W9-BNU-139

A BITTER PILL

# A BITTER PILL

## HOW THE

## MEDICAL SYSTEM

## IS FAILING

## THE ELDERLY

JOHN SLOAN, MD

GREYSTONE BOOKS
D&M PUBLISHERS INC.
Vancouver/Toronto/Berkeley

Copyright © 2009 by John Sloan

13 12 11   5 4 3 2

All rights reserved. No part of this book may be reproduced,
stored in a retrieval system, or transmitted, in any form or by any means,
without the prior written consent of the publisher or a license from
The Canadian Copyright Licensing Agency (Access Copyright).
For a copyright license, visit www.accesscopyright.ca or call toll free
to 1-800-893-5777.

Greystone Books
An imprint of D&M Publishers Inc.
2323 Quebec Street, Suite 201
Vancouver BC Canada V5T 4S7
www.greystonebooks.com

Library and Archives Canada Cataloguing in Publication
Sloan, John, 1947–
A bitter pill : how the medical system is failing the elderly / John Sloan
Includes bibliographical references and index.
ISBN 978-1-55365-455-1
1. Older people—Medical care—Canada. 2. Frail elderly—Medical care—Canada.
3. Medical policy—Canada. I. Title.
RC952.S558 2009   362.198'9700971   C2009-904393-9

Editing by Nancy Flight
Copy editing by Eve Rickert
Text design by Heather Pringle
Cover photograph © Image Source
Printed and bound in Canada by Friesens
Printed on acid-free paper that is forest friendly
(100% post-consumer recycled paper) and has been processed chlorine free
Distributed in the U.S. by Publishers Group West

We gratefully acknowledge the financial support of the Canada Council
for the Arts, the British Columbia Arts Council, the Province of British Columbia
through the Book Publishing Tax Credit, and the Government of Canada through the
Book Publishing Industry Development Program (BPIDP) for our publishing activities.

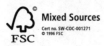

Mixed Sources
Cert no. SW-COC-001271
© 1996 FSC
FSC

# Contents

FOREWORD   1

PREFACE   3

INTRODUCTION   5

1   **The Fragile Elderly**   13
All the Wrong Stuff

2   **Pseudoscience**   39
Where One-Size-Fits-All Health Care Comes From

3   **Poisonous Prevention**   60
Just Keep Takin' Them Pills

4   **Three Blind Dice**   82
Examples of Prevention as a Gamble

5   **The Cathedrals of Crisis**   96
Rescue and the Hospital

6   **Falling Between the Cracks**   116
Geriatric NIMBYism

7   **You Should See the Other Guy**   134
The System in Trouble

8   **Lock Them Up and Throw Away the Key**   158
The Villains of the Piece

9   **Nobody Asked Us**   181
What Fragile Old People Want and Need

10   **Starting Back**   206
Healthier Health Care

EPILOGUE   236

ACKNOWLEDGMENTS   238

REFERENCES   241

INDEX   247

A BITTER PILL

## Foreword

"MAN NEVER LIVES in a state of nature," wrote Simone de Beauvoir. "In his old age, as at every other period of his life, his status is imposed upon him by the society to which he belongs." In *A Bitter Pill* John Sloan depicts the low state to which postindustrial North America has reduced many of our old people, particularly the ones he accurately describes as the "fragile elderly."

Our very word "elderly" is a giveaway: it defines an entire age group by their chronology rather than by their place in the social order. In previous times and in other cultures they would have been called "elders"—that is, human beings with wisdom and experience who fulfilled an honored role in the life of their communities. Today's elderly are seen as has-beens, as a burden, excluded from active life and often isolated even from their families. These are the people Dr. John Sloan cares for, visiting them in their homes, monitoring their health status, working to keep them as functional as possible, and, with distressing frequency, witnessing how they are failed by the medical system—despite his own best efforts.

Sloan is a keen and compassionate observer, and anyone concerned with the care of old people needs to learn from him. He argues, perhaps too generously, that our medical practices work well for younger people with single, identifiable illnesses, but he is, lamentably, on-target in pointing out how inadequate our skills and knowledge base are when it comes to the elderly. "The medical system is set up to help people," he writes, "but it does the opposite for most of the people I look after." His insights about the nature of the vulnerable elderly are textbook precise and, in fact, need to be incorporated in textbooks. He not only recognizes their commonly shared frailties but also acknowledges that *"the frail elderly are different from one another in all sorts of ways."* This willingness to see his geriatric patients not as generic collections of symptoms but as individuals with unique personalities and unique needs is Sloan's greatest strength as a clinician and also as a writer.

Another strength is his ability to question medical orthodoxy, combined with the courage to do so. In today's world prescription drugs make up much of what we physicians offer people by way of treatment and prevention—a sorry fact that reflects our narrowness of perspective and, as well, the overweening influence of the pharmaceutical industry over medical practice. Although Dr. Sloan accepts that "drugs can be really good for people and make them function and feel better," he expresses a healthy skepticism about the widespread use of medications for the prevention of illness among the elderly.

In this, as in all aspects of this indispensable book, what comes across is Sloan's combination of intuition, commitment, rigorous science, and humanity—and, to use a word entirely outside the realm of usual medical discourse, his *love* for a largely ignored, misunderstood, and neglected segment of our society. A segment, we need to recall, we may all join someday.

Gabor Maté, MD
Author of *When the Body Says No: The Cost of Hidden Stress* and *In the Realm of Hungry Ghosts: Close Encounters with Addiction*

# Preface

THIS IS A book about elderly people. Late life is not often an easy time, and I've written this book to describe how I believe it could be easier if we understood it differently. We who do medical care for the elderly could do it much better than we do, and I want people who care for the elderly to understand how we could do that if we could do it together. In this book I'm talking mostly to caregivers, but if you are an elderly person experiencing problems with independence and your medical care, please read this as though it were addressed directly to you. The ideas apply equally to old people caring for themselves.

The majority of older people are women. When I refer to the whole group, I've tended to be inconsistent in whether I call them male or female. Sometimes I just use the plural ungrammatically because it seems easier. I hope my readers will forgive this.

I've included stories about real people in my medical practice, many of whom are still alive. I have tried to disguise the identities of many of the people in these stories. I've sometimes changed names, race, gender, age, and social circumstances while trying to maintain the unique feeling of their situation and our relationship.

I apologize if any readers think they recognize themselves or someone else, especially if they find my description harsh or disapproving. In many of my stories I exaggerate a little for emphasis. Although I often characterize people frankly, I do not intend to be unkind, and I know everyone understands that not being perfect is common to all of us.

The References section provides the titles of a few books, articles, or Web sites that might help an interested reader look a little further into certain subjects. In the interest of simplicity, I haven't referenced these in the text. The Internet or a local library may be useful; thousands of books and Web sites cover the subjects in this book. I would be happy to hear from readers and will help if I can. My e-mail address is tosloan@shaw.ca; my telephone number is (604) 878-4888.

# Introduction

Eighty-six-year-old Mary McCarthy had gotten out of the big-city hospital three days ago. When I visited her in her quiet, dark house, I had trouble hiding my shock.

The last time I had seen Mary, I had wondered if she really needed a house call. In my home care practice I'm used to smell, mess, and rotten food in the fridge. But Mary's house was always spotless, and any aroma was of fresh-cut flowers from her garden. I always had to be careful making suggestions about her health, knowing she was ready and game for an argument (which she usually won). And Mary McCarthy was an attractive woman. I say this from a position of clinical detachment, but it was the truth. She lived a life full of excitement, even though she was old and a lot slower than she used to be.

But this person I confronted three days out of the hospital wasn't going to be getting excited about anything. And she would be lucky to get up onto her feet, let alone pick flowers in her garden. She just sat, slumped in her robe, propped up by pillows, staring at the TV in the corner of the living room. I couldn't tell whether she knew I was there. The curtains were drawn, and a night-light flickered in the corner. I turned to her daughter, Gwen, who gave me a complicated look that said, among other things, *help!*

Six weeks previous, Gwen had called me at about 9 PM because Mary was suddenly short of breath, and I had had a familiar argument with myself. I'm a doctor who looks after older people at home. Going to see if I can figure out what is wrong and then treating it is my job and my commitment. But nine times out of ten, with shortness of breath, we would need a cardiogram, x-rays, and blood tests to be sure we made the right diagnosis. All of these are available that time of night only at the hospital, and the treatment might also involve some things that couldn't be done as well at home. I knew that someone like Mary could probably withstand the treatment she might get at the hospital. Gwen had called 911 on my advice, and I had gone back to watching *Law and Order*.

Mary had landed in our local teaching hospital, where I don't have admitting privileges, and I hadn't heard anything about her since, which was pretty typical of that hospital. They had told Gwen that her mother had had a heart attack and later that she had heart failure, vascular dementia, osteoporosis, diabetes, high blood pressure, and arthritis. Mary had had every kind of study and test imaginable, said Gwen, who was reassured by each of the many doctors who saw her mother that all these problems could be controlled with medication.

Looking quickly at my patient, who was nodding toward a TV show about making a normal person look like a movie star, I took the card of transparent plastic bubbles Gwen handed me. In it I saw a week's worth of Mary McCarthy's medication. The card was a special one with extra-large bubbles: thirty pills a day, divided into four daily doses. I walked across the room, opened the curtains, turned off the television, and asked Mary how she was doing.

THE WAY MODERN medical care is usually practiced is all wrong for old people near the end of their lives. Disasters like the story of Mary McCarthy are frequent, and most of the time they don't need to happen.

This book is about who the Mary McCarthys of this world are, what modern medical care has become, why it's wrong for these people, and what we can do about it. The medical system is set up to help people, but it does the opposite for most of the people I look after. Very old people aren't just older versions of themselves when they were middle-aged, and if we persist in pushing the solutions that work not too badly for younger, healthy people at these very different old ones, we will go right on doing them harm—and over the next couple of decades possibly wreck the health care system in the process. Things need to change.

I've been a family doctor for over thirty years, and most of that time I've looked after old people in their homes. For the last fifteen years I've done home care exclusively for the elderly. My patients are the kind that can't get out to see a doctor in an office or a hairdresser in the mall. When they try, the whole family has to be mobilized days in advance. It takes twenty minutes to get from the front door to the back seat of the car and another twenty from there to the waiting room (usually, for some reason, in the pouring rain). Getting undressed and up onto the examining table is as quick and easy as preparing for spaceflight, and getting back down into the wheelchair is as safe as jumping out of a second-storey window.

The doctor (who could have been me fifteen years ago, when I was in an office), doing his or her best against difficult odds, usually wants blood tests and an x-ray, which would happen in a building across the street.

After trying to go and see the doctor in an office a couple of times, most of my elderly patients have given up. You can probably guess what happens next. Understandably worried family members, neighbors, or just somebody delivering groceries gets concerned about an old person with problems who hasn't been to the doctor in a year. And finally the only available solution is a trip to the hospital or to a nursing home, both of them often one-way.

So I go to my patients instead of making them come to me. I'm quite a bit more mobile than they are. I pack my car (old like my patients, but still reliable) with much of the simple stuff that used to be in my office: blood-pressure machine, earwax syringe, needles, lights, dressings, a computer, and a big box of forms and prescription pads. My beeper and cell phone keep me connected, and I make my appointments on a little PDA. I'm very familiar with apartment security intercom systems and a lot better at parallel parking than I used to be.

At the end of my day I check on test results and make phone calls just the way I did in the office, only I do it at home. And at night and on weekends I make sure my beeper is switched on. This is also no different from the way I used to practice out of my suburban storefront, but now my patients, who still tend to get into trouble suddenly and unpredictably at odd hours, really need me to be available. Most of the calls I get can be handled with reassurance and a daytime visit later on; once in a while I have to go out and see someone late at night. But the idea behind making sure my elderly shut-ins can reach me 24/7 is to keep them out of the hospital.

People are impressed with all this: "What a wonderful practice!" Absolutely. But I'm swimming against the stream. Over the years I've become convinced that there is something wrong with how my profession helps the kind of patients I see. Too many times they end up like Mary McCarthy as we saw her, fresh out of the hospital.

Driving around between visits, I've thought this situation over quite a bit, and the cause boils down to the direction medicine and health care have been going, which is *away* from what my patients need. Trying to help troubled people can be complicated, difficult, and confusing. In the face of such a task, it is important to be organized, and we doctors are famous for being organized or overorganized (a state sometimes referred to as obsessive-compulsive). We do business according to a set of scientific rules. But through day after day of trying to meet the needs of my group of patients, I can't escape this huge and scary fact: *for these people, most of the time, the scientific rules of my profession don't work.*

For a while I thought it was just me. It wouldn't be the first time I was on the wrong track. Plus I'm a born skeptic and tend to see the glass as half-empty. But several conversations I had with people whose opinions I respect confirmed my original worry. At breakfast during a clinical conference, I chatted with a professional statistician (who also enjoyed extremely strong coffee), and he agreed. And not only did he agree with my troubled instinct that scientific rules of practice do not work for my patients, but he also said that the logic and the mathematics used in developing scientific rules in medicine are not always strictly correct. I was surprised to meet someone much more skilled in mathematics and logic than I who shared my vague skepticism about science and medicine. Here was a professional number cruncher who also could not see an unbroken logical chain necessarily anchoring individual patients to scientific safety.

The main problem with the health care of the old people I see is that there is a lack of fit between the solutions and programs universally accepted in the medical system and the characteristics of my group of patients.

Chapter 1 describes this elderly patient group, which I will call the "fragile elderly." Fragile elderly people are not just different from middle-aged people—they are *all different from one another*. Every single thing that is useful at predicting what happens to somebody when we do something for them is, with these old folks, variable. Result: you can't predict what's going to happen. And because you can't predict what's going to happen to fragile elderly people, it's very difficult to predict their response to treatment. Overall, these people just aren't similar or fundamentally predictable, psychologically, socially, or biologically, like the rest of us, whom the medical system is designed to benefit.

In Chapter 2 I describe today's medical system, showing how it has gone in the right direction for most people but in the wrong direction for frail old people. The medical system's universally accepted solutions and programs, which are properly scientific, are what an average, younger, healthy person needs to get the best possible result in treating their one illness, whether that's diabetes, cystic fibrosis, or a broken ankle. This chapter aims to provide an understanding of why the concepts critical to modern health care of "average," "healthy," and "one illness" (not to mention youth) fit the fragile elderly like a red formal ball gown fits an average male rhinoceros.

Chapters 3 through 6 deal with what happens when elderly people and best practice—the treatment generally accepted to work best in any health situation—collide. For nearly all of my patients, the two priorities of usual best-practice health care, prevention and rescue, might as well be from another planet. Chapter 3 looks at the first of these priorities and explains why it may be irrelevant for a lot of old people. Chapter 4 offers some examples of prevention gone wrong.

The medical system's second priority, rescue from crisis, has a totally different practical meaning for the fragile elderly than it has for younger people. Rescue and why it doesn't work is the topic of Chapter 5, including some discussion of the ultimate tool in the rescue kit—the hospital—and why hospitals and the fragile elderly are one another's worst nightmare.

When a health care system is designed to do important things that a large and growing group of people don't need and don't benefit from, it isn't surprising that many of those people aren't getting their real needs met. They tend to fall between the cracks. Reasons for and examples of that worrisome situation are described in Chapter 6.

Chapter 7 looks at the other nightmare involved here, the other vehicle in the collision. In giving old people what they *don't* need, we are doing serious damage to something most of us, at some point, *will* need: a functioning medical system that has the resources to meet traditional health care needs, including crisis. You or I or one of our family members might arrive in an ambulance at the emergency room one night and find it full of eighty- and ninety-year-olds who can't benefit from being there. That is what happens when we try to make the system do what it can't.

In Chapter 8, I consider how health care in the Western world has reached the state it is in. Among the usual characters within that enterprise are several popular targets for blame: doctors, the drug industry, and the health care industry in general. All of them regularly come in for a bucketful of vitriol from other people in the medical system, politicians, and the media. "If only we didn't have to worry all the time about the bottom line, audits, and the priorities of business and bureaucracy." "If only the greedy drug industry weren't constantly shoving medication down our throats." "If only doctors and hospitals would quit thinking about everything as a *disease*." These are the kinds of simple ideas I frequently hear.

Maybe the most distressing of the troubles I experience in the interface between the medical system and my patients is that we somehow just don't *listen* to what frail old people are saying, to what *they* tell us their needs are. I find it easy to fall into this kind of deafness myself. For me, one of the most unappealing characteristics of modern health care is that we ignore what elderly people want. In Chapter 9, I consider what old people are trying to say to us and how we can listen better.

A lot of the problems I describe throughout these chapters arise because my patients and the best-practice health care system miss one another by miles all the time. In Chapter 10, I set down my ideas for what we need to do about that. Mainly, we must learn to see people as individuals, not populations or even members of a population. What is best for this old man is what will work for *him*, individually. What is best for that old lady might not work for anybody else on earth.

The fix for the poor fit that results in bad care for the elderly requires a fundamental, honest change of heart. Tinkering around the edges of the medical system, which we have been doing for decades, won't help. Anyone close to a fragile elderly person (and there will be more and more of us in the next couple of decades) understands that solutions to their problems really matter and are needed *now*. The medical system will change for the better when we all need and want it to badly enough. In the meantime, if I can turn a few minds in the direction of working out individual solutions for individual people, I'll be happy.

# 1 The Fragile Elderly
## All the Wrong Stuff

**PICK ANY THREE**

Here are quick snapshots of three people from my practice, to give you an idea of how different they are from one another.

### ONE: ELLEN GORTON

Ever since I had known Mrs. Ellen Gorton, she had told me she couldn't walk. She got around the house in an old wheelchair. The reasons she gave for why she couldn't walk were always the same: she was tired, her knees ached, she was dizzy, she felt shaky all over, it was the medication. Doctoring each of these in turn didn't make any difference. Stopping any medication made things worse. Treating her as depressed, with medication again, made things worse ("These pills make me tired, make my knees ache, make me dizzy, make me shaky all over"). When I tested her memory, it was pretty close to perfect—she never had any problem remembering and reminding me of the things I had promised to do the last time I saw her. The last time I was there, she had dropped a bomb by telling me she didn't really want to walk and preferred to stay in her wheelchair. She was tremendously overweight, even though she told me she ate nothing but raw vegetables, and that only once a day.

Visiting her was an adventure in other ways. Her son worked all day, but occasionally I saw her daughter-in-law, who was very charming but didn't believe in housekeeping. The house was comprehensively filthy. The whole backyard was destroyed by two dogs to a tin-can-littered dirt pile. One, a black border collie–type pooch, would trot around benignly sniffing here and there, but the other, a brown rottweiler-style killer, would eyeball me very carefully as I came and went, crossing the yard from the lane. I would distract him with a falsetto, "Hello, doggie, nice doggie, there's a good doggie." One day, in a certain mood after spending time with Mrs. Gorton, I did my doggie act as I braved it through the backyard, but, once I got safely outside the gate, I leaned back over the fence, bared my teeth, and growled and barked at him. He ran straight at the gate and slammed into it. Next time he will tear off my leg.

## TWO: HOWARD MCKENZIE

I pulled up a winding driveway, past Japanese gardeners, the smell of fresh-trimmed lawn in the air, to the huge brick house where Joan and Howard McKenzie lived. It was the most expensive neighborhood in town. Howard was in the last stages of Parkinson's disease, and the previous week he had nearly died because his blood pressure was so low he stopped taking liquids. Joan had told me he'd been sleepy. I'd known him for about four weeks and had discovered the low blood pressure on my second visit. It wasn't that easy to convince Joan that the dose of Parkinson's medicine might now be too high, because he had lost a lot of weight, and some of his liver and kidney function, in the last couple of years. "But it was set up by David Hughes," said Joan, looking at me over her French half-glasses as she named the local professor and chief of neurology. Shouldn't Howard be checked by him again? Getting poor Howard out for anything meant an ambulance and quite a bit of sedation. I did convince a specialist to see someone at home about ten years before, but he was a very good friend, and it only happened once.

So Joan and I agreed to try cutting back the dose. I said I would call Dr. Hughes but knew perfectly well he'd return my call when Maui froze over or he got back from Switzerland, whichever was later. Howard didn't participate in this conversation, silently squirming and drooling in his wheelchair. He was busy pulling at the tablecloth and wet handkerchiefs in his lap. Three hovering home support workers moved in to fluff up his pillow and clean up the drool as I headed for the door.

### THREE: GUENTER HAUPTMANN

Running late, I got past the broken apartment entry phone on a low-class high-rise and went up twenty-five floors on the elevator to see Guenter Hauptmann for the first time. Appearing in a dirty bathrobe, he could barely open the door of his apartment. He said, and I could see, that he was almost too weak to stand up. Home care nurses had indicated in their faxed referral that he had gotten out of the hospital several weeks before, after some surgery. I now discovered that everything had been fine until the last ten days, when he had begun to get short of breath and generally feel like hell. His one-room apartment was cluttered. One wall was a giant window overlooking a view of the beach and ocean that made me dizzy. Everything I could see screamed confusion and disorder: upset medication bottles spilling multiple pills, dark wet stains on the bed, the tiny kitchen cluttered and stinking. And he was in congestive heart failure.

I got him some clean, cold water. Nothing I said or did convinced him that he needed to go to the hospital: he flat-out refused and made a terrifyingly pathetic attempt at fighting with me when I tried to lead him to the door. I sat and tried to reason with him for forty minutes, getting more and more behind schedule: nothing doing. So I warned him again and called the pharmacy to try to set up blister packs, including treatment for heart failure and suspected pneumonia.

There was no answer when I tried to raise the apartment manager. I started the process of contacting the home care nurse (who had discharged him two weeks before; at that time he was not in bad shape) and arranged to get back and see Guenter first thing the next day. I considered calling the police but knew they—quite properly—couldn't help. I decided to try to reach family members if I could find out who they were. I hoped to God he would still be alive the next day and possibly a bit better. I had mixed feelings as I punched the elevator button.

*Postscript:* the apartment manager let himself in that night when Guenter didn't answer the door. He was unconscious. The manager called an ambulance, and Guenter was admitted to hospital. He died the next day.

THE CIRCUMSTANCES OF these three people are typical and not typical. That they are individual, are sometimes bizarre, and lack order is typical. But for those same reasons, *there is no typical.* As I describe in this chapter what in geriatrics we call "frailty," it should become clear that in trying to be scientific about people like my patients, we are herding cats.

First I have to deal with some terminology. I'm not sure where "frail" came from, but today it's a universally understood term in health care for the geriatric population made up of people like the three patients I've just described. I don't think it is a bad term; it might evoke "fragile" and "ailing," but it also has a kind of country-style robustness. But "frail" has a specific meaning for a doctor or other health professional, and geriatric social workers or occupational therapists know that "frail" carries a set of operational meanings that help them work efficiently and bring along the correct tools. But to avoid condescension or ageism, I'm not going to use it. Much.

Another frequently used term is "dependent." A widely accepted classification in geriatrics refers only to very frail people as dependent. This seems a misnomer to me, because really everybody I look after is dependent on other people for help every day. It's part of the definition. They might need help with their finances, their transportation, or just about everything in their life, but the bottom line is they need help. Another problem with "dependent" is that everybody is dependent; I'm not very good at flying an airplane, for example. So where does "dependent" start and stop? So I'll try to avoid "dependent" for fear of another kind of misunderstanding.

Nearly everybody I look after is old. The average age of patients in my practice is 83.5, and that average is pulled down by quite a few mentally retarded people I see who are housebound, aged between about 18 and 50. Here we run into another little piece of health care linguistics: nobody ever says "old." It's "elderly." This term gives me the same problems as calling a nursing home a "facility" or a beer a "beverage." Somebody is trying to disguise a reality and thinks it can be done using a high school thesaurus. My solution to that problem will be to use "old" and "elderly" interchangeably. We're just referring to chronological age, which (whether you interpret the high numbers as meaning someone is decrepit or wonderfully seasoned) seems a reasonably neutral fact.

One of the most consistent things about my patients is that it doesn't take much to cause them problems. For this reason, my favored modifier in describing them is "fragile." Thus, when I generalize about the people I am talking about in this book, I will usually use "fragile elderly" or "fragile old people." "Fragile" means about the same as "frail." Conventional medical care is fine for people who are not part of the group but is wrong for everyone else. But who is included in this group? At what point should we switch to the different medical care I'm advocating?

Who is frail and who isn't has been thought and written about over many years by many well-informed academics. There are scales of frailty, which grade function from almost no impairment to very severely impaired. It has been shown that an older person's grade on a scale of this kind lines up with how long she is probably going to live and her chances of ending up in a nursing home. There is a certain self-fulfilling character to this: naturally, the older and sicker someone is, the worse they will tend to do in the future, no matter where they fall on some scale. But, probably for some pretty good reasons, a lot of time and energy has gone into developing frailty definitions.

The academic authors who have studied scales of frailty and worked with mathematical models to try to develop predictive tools don't seem to me to give us a cut-off point that will tell us exactly when we should change our approach to care. The Canadian geriatrician Kenneth Rockwood, one such well-known academic author, tells us about one scale of frailty: "Applying the

Clinical Frailty Scale to patients requires judgment. The fabric of individual health has many strands, and it seems likely that some clinicians sometimes used factors not precisely specified in our brief set of descriptors."

Many strands indeed. The truth is that everyone working with fragile elderly people understands that at some point in each person's life the solutions offered by modern scientific medical care don't work anymore. I wonder, in fact, if part of the reason we insist on conventional medical care way beyond when it is still working is that we're uncomfortable about being unable to say just when it isn't anymore. For me that isn't such a big problem. There is no academic definition of the fragile or frail elderly, and that's just fine.

So who is "fragile" (frail) in the sense that I mean here? To whom does the quite different approach to health care I'm trying to sell apply? Well, I have an answer for you. The most important definition of fragility or frailty *is the definition the person makes for herself.* Because many fragile old people are unable to make decisions for themselves, you, the caregiver, may be the one to decide. The process may be collaborative between the two of you. But the point in an old person's life at which she changes from conventional medical care to something different is when she or her decision makers choose to. Once that choice is made, she steps into the last adventure of her life.

A fragile elderly person may be an eighty-two-year-old lady who has always driven her car, made decisions for herself, and done her own cooking. All of a sudden she can't drive anymore and is having trouble taking a bath. You could be the middle-aged kids of someone whose memory has gotten bad enough that she can't keep the place clean anymore, long ago gave up managing her money, and now is resisting help with getting dressed in the morning, even though she obviously needs it. Someone considering a change in his health care might be a tough-minded, self-reliant semihermit who has just run out of steam and needs help holding life together. The point is that it's the elderly person, with the best advice available and maybe through a substitute decision maker, who has to decide when to leave behind the conventional medical system's prevention-and-rescue agenda.

But crossing that line into being a fragile elderly person doesn't mean giving up, except giving up some things that are now pretty well useless. It just means that the priorities are going to change. Forget visits to the cardiologist every six weeks to make sure your preventive medication is exactly correct. Throw away the hospital parking pass that enables visiting the osteoporosis specialist who makes sure the bone density is okay. Quit the visits to the fussy family physician, which result in two new medications and three referrals to clinical boutiques in hospitals and specialty centers, which leads to a round of appointments, blood tests, pharmacy and nutrition consultations, and swallowing assessments. The good news is, a fragile old person might actually have some time to herself!

Certain characteristics define the fragile elderly, for whom conventional medical care is no longer useful, and those characteristics are also important in making decisions about what kind of care they *should* receive.

The first characteristic of the fragile elderly is that *they have multiple pathology*—that is, they have lots of illnesses or health conditions.

People get more illnesses as they get older, though this is one of those generalities to which there are lots of exceptions. Some newborn babies have a large number of terrible things the matter with them, and at the other end of life, some people well into their nineties have never been sick a day in their life. But on average, as time goes by, people accumulate health problems. "Multiple pathology" is what geriatrics professionals call this. A typical medical chart on one of my patients reads like the *Merck Manual*.

The second characteristic of the fragile elderly is that *they are dependent on others for activities of daily living.*

Eventually, all the health problems these people have cause trouble. The main causes of dependence are that they can't remember, so they can't organize and plan, or they can't walk, so they lose the ability to get around.

Memory trouble usually comes from dementia, which can cause people to lose a lot more than their memory. Alzheimer's disease is the most famous cause of dementia, but you can become demented from all sorts of other causes. Most of the common dementias get worse over time. And in spite of the optimism that existed thirty or forty years ago in the early days of geriatrics, very few dementias are reversible. Thus, people with memory problems need some help in managing their lives because they can't organize or plan and eventually can't think very well about anything at all. About half the people in my practice have some dementia.

The other big group of dependent people are the ones who can't get around, or can't get around safely, or take forever to get from A to B. This difficulty occurs for a variety of reasons. Many such patients have had strokes, and so one side of their body is paralyzed or their movements are uncoordinated. Another cause is arthritis, usually from wearing away of joints, which means it hurts when they stand up, walk, or maneuver. Some days it seems that nearly everybody I see is in pain, and pain has a long list of causes besides arthritis. But one consistent thing about pain: it really slows people down, no matter what the

cause. Then there are people who are just physically weak all the
time, and it can be very hard to find out the cause of that. Just
about any illness, many drugs, deconditioning (two weeks of sitting in a chair doing nothing, for example), and depression are
some of the things that make old patients weak. As a result, they
can't stand up or get around, and they need help managing the
activities of daily life: they are dependent. Some have trouble doing such activities as brushing their teeth, taking a shower, using a toilet, getting dressed, and eating a meal. Such people are
usually housebound and have trouble shopping, keeping a place
clean, doing their banking, planning and cooking meals, getting
around the community, using a telephone, doing the laundry,
and taking medication.

Daily living activities typically collapse in sequence. At first
an elderly person can't quite do her finances or drive her car
safely anymore. Later she has trouble taking a bath and getting
dressed. Eventually she may need help just eating.

The patients described at the beginning of this chapter are
at different stages of dependence. Mrs. Gorton is stuck in her
wheelchair and can't do anything that requires walking around.
She cannot get out of the house without three or four strong dog-
friendly people to get her down the stairs. Luckily, so far she is
able to boost her great weight from the wheelchair to the toilet
and back and also to get in and out of bed. But someone has to
help her with shopping, getting to the bank, and doing the laundry. She also needs help taking a bath or shower. She is still pretty
sharp mentally, however, and her memory is intact. So she can
still perform intelligence- and memory-based activities. She can
take her medication, can make and answer a phone call, and, although she claims she eats her vegetables raw, could safely rustle

up a pot of cardboard-box mac and cheese on top of the stove or heat up a TV dinner in the oven.

Mr. McKenzie is at the heavy end of dependence and needs pretty much total care for everything, including eating. His disease has long ago taken away his ability to communicate, let alone to consider and be involved in any decisions about his life.

And finally, Guenter Hauptmann was in a whole different type of trouble when I saw him: he was in crisis. Guenter couldn't do much of anything for himself, but he had got that way quickly. What was he like before he had his surgery? Everything I could find out told me he had been only mildly dependent. After the surgery he needed more help for a short time but then seemed to be improving.

I am not that happy about my performance with Mr. Hauptmann. A doctor looking after that type of patient has to analyze a crisis, figure out what kind of action is possible and reasonable, and take it using whatever resources are available. What could I or should I have done? I'm not sure.

Once somebody can't do a basic life activity anymore, they're dependent for that activity. But life can carry on without a huge amount of trouble as long as someone who is dependent has all of his needs met. Where there is an unmet need, there's going to be a problem. Sometimes the problem progresses slowly, as when an apartment gets filthier and filthier (the way some of my patients' homes smell can make me gag), or when somebody slowly loses weight because he's only eating every couple of days. Other times the problem develops more quickly and may become a crisis, as when someone spends three days in bed with no food or water or access to a toilet. People who can't manage for themselves must have their daily needs met by someone else.

It is also important to make sure the problem can't be fixed (or to fix it if it is fixable, of course). This means that some capable attention must be focused on the person. Traditionally, dependent elderly people would be referred to a geriatrics specialist or sent to a geriatric evaluation and management unit. Either way experienced, skilled practitioners (perhaps a team including a social worker, a nurse, a rehabilitation professional, a doctor, and possibly a pharmacist) go over such people's problems, medications, supports, and so on and tune them up so that the patients are in the best possible shape they can be in. Success of this tune-up is measured by performance at daily living activities. And so, out of the other end of this comprehensive evaluation and treatment come some people who are doing a lot better (maybe they drive away in their car, say) and another group whom we can call fragile because we're sure their problems are not remediable.

The third characteristic of the fragile elderly is that *daily function is a number-one priority.*

Getting through each day is so important to a fragile elderly person that it becomes (or it should become) a defining priority. In such a person's daily life, there often isn't anything as important as function, which means being able to do the things she needs to get through that day, with or without somebody helping her. This is one of the main ideas I'm offering in this book: best-practice health care is what modern medicine has to give the fragile elderly—often all it has to give. But because of the importance of daily living function in people like my patients, best-practice health care comes in a way-distant second place to supporting their daily needs.

I gave a presentation at a conference a couple of years ago and was lucky enough to be joined by a good friend of mine who is an academic geriatric doctor. Our subject was how much textbook preventive medical care we should be offering to our patients. We took different points of view, partly to keep the audience from going to sleep. My friend and I are philosophically quite similar: we both believe that we must do the best we can for our patients and that everybody is different. But he comes from the internal medicine side of geriatric care, so he gets a refresher course in the catechism of prevention every time he talks to his colleagues, and this is what he focuses on. And in a way I agree with him. But I believe function is a first priority, though not the only thing worth thinking about. My academic geriatric friend is focused on prevention, and I don't have any problem with that as long as the priorities are straight. According to his set of rules, we should treat fragile elderly people using evidence-based guidelines and *then* see whether they are functioning independently up to their potential. Then if the guidelines have to be modified to get best possible function, that's okay with him. But I see the priorities differently.

Rules of practice that emphasize prevention might be useful to any one fragile elderly patient, but keeping that person independent by improving or supporting her function is always absolutely useful. That is why I think function is a top priority. No question, if a very elderly person is walking as well as she possibly can and living a convenient and adequately supported life, and if practical plans are in place for what is probably going to go wrong in the future, then it makes sense to try to ensure that she has normal blood pressure, normal cholesterol, and reasonable control of her high blood sugar. But the moment any treatment or drug given to achieve these theoretical benefits gets in the way of keeping her on her feet or puts her at serious risk for drug side effects or other trouble, the theoretical stuff goes into the garbage chute. Function comes first.

The fourth characteristic of the fragile elderly is that *crisis for them is always a crisis of function.*

The fragile elderly get into trouble regularly. Most often the trouble they get into involves a relatively minor health problem, but a lack of function turns the minor problem into a crisis. We respond, however, most often with the resources and tools the medical system has developed for rescue in an emergency. But again, function should be the priority.

Guenter Hauptmann was an exceptional case of crisis. He was in the unusual situation among fragile old people where pushing the critical care panic button might have saved his life, if only he had let me. That said, if he had had responsible care at home, he might never have got as far into trouble as he was, the illness would have been recognized early, and it probably could have been treated at home. I like to imagine that if I had been seeing him for the tenth time, not the first, things might have turned out differently.

Exceptions aside, for most of my patients crisis usually isn't a serious health problem. And when it is, it usually isn't a serious health problem that will respond to critical care treatment. Rather, it tends to be a fairly minor problem such as a urinary tract infection, a fall that bruises your backside, a new medication, losing 10 percent of your strength, or four days of diarrhea. These are typical examples of the kinds of things that result in crisis of function. None of them needs any medical rocket science. But because each of them can stop an old person cold with sudden loss of independence, that person needs quick, comprehensive daily living support and good primary medical care at home.

In a crisis the medical task is to be sure it isn't a Guenter Hauptmann–type situation, make a tentative diagnosis, start simple treatment if necessary, and be careful not to make things worse. If a sudden crisis of function does turn out to be the kind of thing we all usually think of as a crisis (a heart attack, a broken bone, something ruptured inside the stomach), or if it looks as if it might be such a thing, it's time to pull everyone together and have a thoughtful conversation. Family, friends, nurses, the doctor—anyone who is part of the old person's world—can help balance the risks of enduring the illness at home against the risks of being in the hospital, remembering always that chances are hospital treatment won't change the outcome much.

Ideally this conversation will have taken place in advance. What is needed in a crisis of function is support of function and keeping medical care effective but simple.

The fifth defining characteristic of the fragile elderly is that *comfort is an overriding priority.*

Although function has to be pretty close to the top of the priority list, comfort should stand beside it as another overriding priority in treatment. Comfort just means absence of misery—physical, psychological, or social. Textbook preventive treatment should only be considered if it improves or at least does not hinder comfort.

One of the most grotesquely disturbing situations I see, especially when old people are in hospital, is the grim sacrifice of comfort in favor of the medical system's priorities of rescue and prevention. Walking along a hospital hallway not long ago, I saw a very old man being wheeled on a stretcher into the MRI suite. Even knowing nothing at all about his circumstances, I knew that the psychological and physical misery I could see on his face, and what he was about to experience while his insides were being imaged, very likely wouldn't bring him any benefit. We are, I suppose, socialized to sacrifice in the name of modern health care, just as a religious person might give up something important in the service of their belief. But making a sacrifice in the service of religion usually provides a benefit. Grinning and bearing the misery of cookbook health care usually does no such thing for the fragile old people swallowing dozens of pills and trucking around the community and hospitals receiving our sacrament-like investigation and treatment.

The sixth characteristic of the fragile elderly, and a very important one, is that *the fragile elderly are different from one another in all sorts of ways.*

My patients are not only different from younger people—they are also different from one another. At the start of this chapter I suggested that trying to be scientific about fragile old people is like herding cats and tends to prevent us from coming up with a satisfactory general definition of frailty. This waywardness, a tendency to be different from one another, is a big part of what makes these people the way they are. In other words they are heterogeneous, or diverse, and this heterogeneity makes a huge difference to drug treatment and to how we need to think about these people in general. A huge difference.

Let's look at a concrete example: kidney function. Kidney function is important to drug treatment, because many drugs are filtered out by the kidneys and gotten rid of in the urine. Drugs do the good things they are supposed to do only once you get enough in your bloodstream. But the catch, of course, is that the more drug you get into your bloodstream, the more you run into the *bad* things that drugs sometimes do, the so-called side effects. The hope is that there exists a sort of ideal blood level for each drug where the good things have started to happen and the bad ones haven't yet. How much drug is in the blood at any time depends (if the drug is one of the ones that the kidneys filter out) on how well the kidneys are working.

Young people tend to have really good kidney function, and it doesn't vary very much: your twenty-year-olds (and forty-five-year-olds) all tend to have about the same kidney filtering function. But as you get older, particularly when you get really old, two things happen. One, kidney function gets worse. So an average eighty-year-old patient will absolutely have worse kidney function than she did when she was twenty. But thing number two is that the older you get, the wider the *range* of kidney function gets. Kidney function becomes heterogeneous. Result: blood levels of kidney-filtered drugs are heterogeneous. No surprise. One elderly person has kidney function close to that of a normal forty-year-old; another one has awful, barely functioning kidneys. Give a kidney-filtered drug at its textbook dose to the first one, everything is cool. Give it to the second one, the blood level is through the roof and side effects have her flat on her back.

The liver is another organ that looks after blood levels of active drugs. It changes drugs into inactive forms, but, like the kidneys, it does that at a reasonably predictable rate—in young people. In the elderly it's the same story as with the kidneys: liver function is all over the place.

And so it goes with just about everything biological that determines what happens when we give a drug to an old person. And none of these things are related to one another. Your grandmother might have great kidneys but almost no liver function. Or she could have trouble with both. So how are we going to decide how much medication to give her? This is a tough question, the non-answer to which is coming up in a minute.

I called the first characteristic of the fragile elderly multiple pathology. There are exceptions, but fragile elderly people tend to have lots of health problems. Even when you're dealing with a doctor like me who hates medication (I don't really—what I hate is the wrong medication at the wrong time for the wrong person), and even when the doctor has his or her priorities straight, having a lot of health problems means being on a lot of medication. "Priorities straight" means prescribing as I believe we always should for patients like mine: only to help with comfort and function. There are a lot of health conditions that make people miserable and prevent them from doing what they need to do, which medication can help.

I'm going to give three examples of when drugs work, but there are dozens. Being in pain has to be one of the worst things in the world. I use drugs that are effective for pain a lot, because making somebody's pain go away is worth paying a price for. Codeine, for example, can work really well for some middling-level pain, but it can make some people constipated and woozy. So is it worth taking laxatives and living with the wooziness not to be in pain? Many people say yes.

Most of the drugs I use for depression work. And being depressed, feeling sad, and not getting any pleasure out of anything is horrible, as anyone who's experienced it can tell you. Three weeks after starting the medication, in spite of the side effects and changes to other drugs that may be necessary, a hopelessly unhappy old person wakes up one morning glad for the first time in months that the sun is shining. It may be the sixth drug that person is on, which may make their medical care pretty complicated. Is seeing the world on the bright side again worth it? Again, most of the time that's a yes.

Parkinson's disease causes people to slow down and stiffen up and has a big impact on function. There is effective treatment. The drugs are very biologically active, and they have side effects, just like most other worthwhile medicines. If I can manage to keep one eye on the patient's walking better, because the Parkinson's stiffness and slowness improves, and the other eye on the famous side effects, it's possible to strike a bargain with this class of drugs—temporarily, at least. Does the good outweigh the bad? Usually for a while.

Drugs can really be good for people and make them function and feel better.

Gathering the characteristics we have so far, our old folks look like a group of people with a lot of health problems, who are dependent on others for daily activities, for whom function and a functional approach to crisis are important, for whom comfort is a priority, and who are very different from one another. And it happens that they are usually on quite a bit of medication.

This is important, because of the seventh characteristic of the fragile elderly: *their response to medication is unpredictable.*

There are two kinds of medicines in the world: those that make you feel better now and those that prevent a bad event in the future. A painkiller would be one of the first kind; a cholesterol-lowering drug one of the second. How do we tell whether each of these kinds of drugs is working? Well, with the first kind the answer is right in your face thirty minutes after you take the pill. Either you feel better or you don't. With the second it's a little more complicated. You have to trust that somebody or something knows what's going on and is giving you good advice. It's with these on-faith preventive drug treatments that the fragile elderly really start running into problems.

Because biological functions vary so much from one old person to another, *when you give a fragile elderly person any medication, you have no idea what's going to happen.*

This uncomfortable, potentially frightening truth comes up every day in my practice and for any doctor prescribing drugs to an old person. How can you prescribe when you don't know what's going to happen? Well, complications and unanswered questions are just facts of life. This applies to every prescription written for any fragile old person.

If we really don't have much idea what medication is going to do, prescribing for the elderly has to be very different than it would be if we could make confident predictions. Any prescribing doctor who believes that unpredictability can be overcome by prescribing according to usual guidelines is dreaming. Even if we could properly measure kidney and liver function in older people, even if there were ways of estimating things like protein, fat, volume, and receptor dynamics in each of them, most prescribing goes on against a background of several other medications the person is already taking, so you can easily get all sorts of unpredictable drug interactions. When we write prescriptions for the fragile elderly, we need a different kind of science from the kind practiced in drug studies.

Any attempt to give old people a cookbook regimen of treatment is doomed. The fragile elderly on drugs need to be watched carefully. And, especially for people who have trouble getting out to go to a doctor's office, a vigilant home care family doctor is about the only person in a position to do that.

Heterogeneity produces unpredictability. Old people are different from one another, so we don't know in advance what drugs will do to them. That unpredictability also applies to other things. How much indignity will someone put up with, how will she feel about being cleaned after a bowel movement by someone she's never met before, how much reassurance does she need, and how tactful and reasonable will she be about, say, money? I can't see much point in trying to predict in advance what a fragile old person's response will be to things like home care, help with finances, a friendly visitor, or a daughter being out of town.

Defining characteristic number eight of the fragile elderly is that *illnesses don't look the way the textbook says they should.*

Unpredictability goes one step further when we look at what happens when an elderly person gets sick. Mr. Hauptmann had pneumonia, but instead of a fever, cough, and chest pain, as you would expect in that disease from reading a textbook of internal medicine, he had weakness and confusion. Another patient of mine had the flu, and, along with the cough and aching we're all familiar with, she too had weakness and confusion.

The older and frailer someone gets, the less likely she is to show a doctor the textbook presentation of any illness. A heart attack shows up as low blood pressure, not chest pain. A urinary tract infection shows up as not being able to hold the urine and getting confused, not burning when you pee. A stroke manifests as falling, not weakness on one side of the body. Et cetera.

The ninth and last characteristic of the fragile elderly is that *they are near the end of their lives.*

The psychological side of life for old people is influenced by their function and the care they get but also by their own understanding of where they are in the course of their lives.

This characteristic of not having much time is a little less conventional, less palatable, and probably more controversial than some of the others. Academic talk on this subject tends to masquerade behind mathematical abstractions. We don't see "Near the End of Her Life" on most textbook lists of characteristics of frailty. But it is one. And it does make a difference to how we ought to be thinking about and helping our patients, clients, neighbors, friends, and loved ones when they are old and need help.

Anyone who meets the definition of a fragile old person doesn't get better but tends to get worse and then die. This isn't pleasant, but it is a hard fact I'm afraid we need to face.

What is that short time usually like for the people living it? Illness has a certain relationship to functional impairment. Because that sounds straight out of a theoretical textbook, I'll illustrate it with a couple of quick real-life stories.

A couple of months ago I woke up with the flu. The flu is an illness, but not a very important one (maybe two on a scale of ten). What was the impact on my function? I'm healthy (touching wood) at a little over sixty, and the impact wasn't much at all. I shouldn't admit it, but I went right on working after grabbing a couple of Tylenol with codeine. Even if I had decided to take it easy, I certainly could have still walked around, made breakfast, and gone out shopping.

Several months earlier I had been called to see Margaret Bellamy, who is eighty-nine and has trouble with the activities of daily life. Mrs. Bellamy weighs in at about ninety pounds and lives alone in a little apartment; she can walk using an aluminum walking frame and can get to the bathroom and back to bed or to her chair. She can dress herself, but it takes forty-five minutes. A lovely immigrant lady comes in and makes her breakfast and gives her her medication every morning. Mrs. Bellamy is a little bit forgetful but is not too bad; daughter number one, who lives twenty minutes away, does the banking and shopping.

One morning Mrs. Bellamy woke up with that same flu I had. She couldn't get out of bed, she was coughing, and she was short of breath. Her bones ached every time she moved, and she was very weak. She couldn't seem to figure out what time it was, and, when her helper rang the entry phone, she couldn't make it over to let her in.

The difference between Mrs. Bellamy and me with this very similar flu is immense. And this is what I meant by the relationship of illness to functional impairment. Two people, same illness. Breathtaking difference in its impact on function. I like to say that somebody like Margaret Bellamy is on the "slippery slope"; a little bit of illness produces a very big, important change in function.

People like my patients start out relatively capable and then decline more or less in a straight line until they die. But this theoretical straight line isn't the real picture, either. Small, unimportant-sounding illnesses, accidents, social changes, and other minor health disturbances come along all the time and have a huge effect on independence and need for help. So life's more or less stable, gradual decline in function is punctuated by sudden, unpredictable changes (suddenly Mrs. Bellamy couldn't get out of bed). Most of the time those changes are temporary.

With Margaret Bellamy, the home support worker called the manager, was let in, and called me, and I went and visited. The agency authorized extra help for a week, and Mrs. Bellamy got her needs seen to and recovered. But sometimes with the medical system we have today, the ending isn't so happy. Crisis may be mismanaged, with unnecessarily ugly results.

In talking about people for whom I care a great deal, I hope that when I say, "decline more or less in a straight line until they die," it doesn't sound as though I'm advocating abandoning caring for them. Keep in mind that everyone dies. We don't know when, but with older, fragile people, we know it's probably pretty soon.

It may help to compare how we think about the fragile elderly with how we think about a group known in health care as "palliative." Palliative patients are typically people expected to die within six months. Traditionally they are mostly cancer patients, but they also include many folks with heart, lung, or other serious diseases nobody can cure. In the palliative-care culture, death and dying are taken to be natural, very real, of course inevitable, and coming up within a clearly defined period of time. With the people I care for at home, death and dying are just as natural, real, and inevitable. The difference has to do with when death is expected.

When we don't know when someone will die, we are afraid of a self-fulfilling prophecy ("Dad's going to die soon anyway, so why would we bother investigating his heart and sending him to a specialist?") or of just being calloused and unfair. But instead of preparing for death, talking about it in a sensitive and forthright way, and focusing on comfort and function, we buy into the taboo on the subject. Death scares most people. And it is particularly upsetting to contemplate talking to somebody else about it, somebody for whom it might be coming along pretty soon, and with whom we may have a complicated, ambivalent relationship, carrying all the baggage of most of a lifetime.

Part of the health care professional mindset is the tendency to put people into pigeonholes. Palliative care patients need their pain controlled, but really we should offer effective pain control to everybody, not just people who qualify as palliative in that they are expected to die in six months and are in a certain program of care. In the same way, we should be thinking of and talking about dying as though it is something natural, inevitable, and eventually acceptable with *everyone*, not just palliative care patients.

But too often with the fragile elderly we don't talk about death—we whisper and tiptoe when the subject comes up, in fact—and so we leave our dear old people, who we can be damn sure are thinking about it, isolated and frightened. Worse, we carry on with the usual health care preoccupation with prevention of and rescue from death. So we end up in a sort of limbo where we are halfhearted about prevention and rescue but not quite prepared to abandon them. We partly excuse ourselves from meeting these people's real needs because after all, we still offer that prevention and rescue, which is good health care, isn't it?

I have talked about dying with hundreds of old people. One thing I'm pretty sure about as a result is that they don't share the prevalent taboo about it. They know it's coming. And so our fear of death itself, and of talking about it, is usually obvious to them and adds to any barriers there may be to communicating effectively with one another, at a time when effective communication is really important.

We don't face the fact that old people are near the end of life in a way that is helpful to them. Nor do we let ourselves fully appreciate that the good time we so wish to provide for our elderly people is not a long time. Because we are making the commitment to provide it for them, I think we're entitled to consider that it won't last forever. If we are to be practical in caring for fragile old people, we need to take all the realities into account.

I hope you now have an idea of how my patients are different from the rest of the world. They are also all different from one another. They have lots of problems. If I've done my job properly, all those problems are taken care of as well as they can be, but they haven't gone away. Because of the problems, my patients can't look after themselves, so they need help. Making sure that they are as well as they can be, to minimize the help they need, and keeping them as comfortable as possible are very important priorities in caring for them. But the amount of help they need can change suddenly, and that kind of change can be a pretty serious disaster. Treatment of these people with drugs is a double-edged sword, with the sharper side pointed at the patient. We are ambivalent about the idea that old people, who are important to us for all sorts of different reasons, only have a short time to live. Because of that we might make their suffering worse without meaning to. The medical system as we find it, far from meeting their needs, sometimes seems preoccupied with avoiding their needs altogether. It is an incredibly complex and compelling situation.

I've said we should be very careful in prescribing medication for fragile old people, should attend primarily to their comfort and function, and should deal with their crises in a creative way. Why aren't we doing these things?

To try to answer that question, in Chapter 2 I will lift the hood on scientific health care, the engine that powers prevention and medical rescue, which are today's health care priorities. Understanding how this magnificent vehicle we have created got to be the way it is might help us appreciate why it is leaving some of its most needy potential passengers at the side of the road.

# 2 Pseudoscience
Where One-Size-Fits-All Health Care
Comes From

## ELIZABETH O'MALLEY

Mrs. O'Malley didn't go to the hospital anymore when she had chest pain. She was ninety-six and had had "heart attack" as a diagnosis on her last three hospital admissions. She had ended up in the hospital because, not wanting to bother me, she called either the apartment manager or the woman next door when she was having trouble. They responded the way every normally socialized member of the public would: they called an ambulance.

Each time, Mrs. O'Malley would come back out of the hospital with standard textbook doses of heart attack–preventing drugs that gave her a very slow heart rate and very low blood pressure. As soon as the admitting doctors saw Mrs. O'Malley's slightly elevated level of troponin in her blood (the gold-standard test for heart attack), they would make the heart attack diagnosis and treat her accordingly. Mrs. O'Malley was one of those people whose troponin level was just high for some obscure biological reason.

None of these hospital specialists would have ever dreamed of calling me. In fairness, they may have been accustomed to not being able to reach family doctors. If I found out Mrs. O'Malley was in the hospital before she got out, there was no way I could reach any of the specialists on the telephone, and if I could have, my argument about past problems probably wouldn't have counted for much compared with the profession's and the hospital's rules of practice.

Once Mrs. O'Malley got home and I very carefully got her back onto the absolutely minute doses of heart attack–preventing medication that she could tolerate, she was fine. One day she may have the kind of heart attack that has a big effect on circulation, and she will probably die quickly of it, maybe even in her sleep.

> Is it not really strange that human beings are normally deaf to the strongest argument while they are always inclined to overestimate measuring accuracies?
>
> ALBERT EINSTEIN, *THE BORN-EINSTEIN LETTERS*

> The central point is that we have created a world we don't understand.
>
> NASSIM NICHOLAS TALEB, *FOOLED BY RANDOMNESS*

MRS. O'MALLEY IS getting what modern health care has to offer: consistent, reliable, scientifically proven, evidence-based preventive care and high-tech rescue from crisis. What is the matter with that? Isn't our health care technology one of the undisputed crowning achievements of civilization? And if it has limitations, aren't very capable people working on them and making progress daily?

I'm sure this is all true. The problems with the medical system have nothing to do with its not being good at what it does or with the people in charge. What it does—and usually does extremely well—is (1) prevent health problems and (2) rescue people who, in spite of prevention, develop health problems. But what modern health care does so well is the wrong thing for people like Mrs. O'Malley.

Why does our old friend Mary McCarthy come out of the hospital ten times worse than when she went in? Is she just an exception, a rare but predictable occurrence that bucks a trend of otherwise unbroken success? My practice is full of Mary McCarthys. Sudden deterioration after getting textbook treatment is a regular event. We keep paying a price for health care's success through its overriding priorities, and the bill gets presented to people like that old lady, at life's end.

The trouble is, I don't think you can constructively criticize a well-entrenched and almost universally credited method without attacking its foundations. Picture me, if you like, trying to keep the powder (my conviction about how we should be looking after old people) dry for the next twenty pages or so. I'm wading, you'll have no trouble imagining, into a river, with my eye on the opposite side. Here be alligators and who knows what else. Shall we wade in a bit deeper?

Somewhere at the bottom of this river is science, with deep roots that go back to ancient Greece, even though its earliest real showing at the surface was around the end of the 16th century. Up to our chins in the current, we will brush up against epidemiology, the science of health care, bottom-feeding a diet of legitimacy from its history of the defeat of infectious diseases. Much more recently this big friendly fish has evolved into an all-consuming predator of pretty well everything else in the water by lending its logic—and that legitimacy—to a fast-moving cousin, the randomized controlled trial.

Farther out in the water and closer to the surface we can see the more ordinary and numerous fish: doctors, physiotherapists, social workers, nurses, people from the health industry, health insurers, and, swimming around trying to keep our noses above the water, health care consumers—patients, clients, adults, whatever we choose to call ourselves. Going down into this fanciful health care river, I imagine, for the third time, would be your typical fragile elderly person from my home care practice.

In we go.

It is easy to believe in the modern medical system. How could anybody not feel gratitude for its stunning accomplishments: cataract and reconstructive joint surgery (they almost never fail), the conquest of cancers with chemotherapy, and the near-magical survival of tiny premature babies. Three examples among dozens.

Unless you live on an island with no TV, radio, or Internet, you will hear the messages modern health care sends, in the way the media interpret them. We are blasted and caressed from all sides with health information based on scientific studies: the dangers of trans fats, the risk of cancer from sunlight (or is it osteoporosis benefit from sunlight?), the risk to children playing with toys made in China. It seems that the public-responsive media have a rule that every half-hour TV news show or morning paper has to tell us about what to do, or keep away from, to not get sick. And in an odd way we love it, don't we? Our appetite can never quite be satisfied.

What's with this fascination with health? It doesn't stop when we turn off the TV. The whole food industry has overturned itself in the interest of health, especially prevention. Just try to get, in a supermarket or a restaurant, a steak, deliciously marbled with fat, that would have met high quality standards in the 1940s. It is practically against the law. There is no way any informed consumer would touch it.

Safety and avoiding injury dominate transportation and the workplace. If you travel at all, you will be familiar with flight attendants' preoccupation with keeping seat belts on and seat backs in their full upright position. Never mind that you're about as likely to survive a real air accident as being chopped into thirty little pieces. I work part-time in a government health department office, and for over a week much of the energy of the unit was directed to learning about the health risks of mouse droppings after one of the little gray creatures was discovered under someone's desk. I'm not joking. You can imagine a world not too far off where smoking a cigarette or riding your bike without full protective armor will be punishable by six months in jail.

I scramble to qualify this. Recklessness where health and safety are concerned is dangerous and should be discouraged. But somewhere between throwing caution to the winds and running your life according to evening news reports of the latest study linking your favorite pastime to a dread disease, there has to be some sort of common sense. Trust me: paying close attention to talk-show traffic isn't going to tell you where that reasonable compromise is.

I sense something a bit furtive in our fascination with health—or is it really fascination with death and disease? We are free to buy what we want, and I wonder if we keep pushing for more and more about health and sickness because we get a perverse thrill from it. The media are only giving us what we choose to consume. Getting sick, getting hurt, and particularly having these things happen insidiously through some process or exposure nobody would ever have suspected as being dangerous are the kind of thing we hate but in a way are secretly eager to hear about. It's the same awful instinct that draws us to the scene of an accident or a house fire and then (if we're brutally honest with ourselves) lets us down when there aren't any victims. Bad news is good news. It's not fair to expect the free media to resist tapping in to that kind of sentiment. And human nature isn't going to change.

A natural connection that probably nobody intended exists between health care "information" and journalism's needs. As a result, health care is in your face whenever you're awake. It's hard to argue that that isn't a good thing, unless you believe, as I do, that modern health care is in certain ways *bad*. Bad, at least, for some people.

Modern health care seems wonderful to us partly because we are told it rests on science. Science is taught to every schoolchild, and most people now consider science as close to an absolute authority as you can get in this world. It almost seems to offer what some of us would otherwise expect from religion. Scientific experts enjoy unquestioned credibility. But what is science, really?

Philosophy of science textbooks tell us that science is a *method*. And the more curious I get about what science really is, the less I find to support the idea that it can give us a satisfying answer to fundamental questions like, What is real? The great pioneers of science in the Enlightenment probably never intended science to be a search for answers to that kind of question. So possibly there isn't a lot of justification for thinking of science as a shortcut to absolute authority.

But isn't it true that one of the strengths of science is its ability to *prove* things? Doesn't it give us an important way to be certain about things? Isaac Newton's predictions about the planets were proven correct by observations through telescopes, right? And those observations were repeated again and again.

Maybe, but then for a short time in the early 20th century the scientific brain trust waited on the edge of its academic chair for the results of measurements that would confirm, or not, predictions by a famously obscure physicist named Albert Einstein. He had come up with the idea that Newton's understanding of the physical universe wasn't the whole story. It turned out his idea fit the measurements perfectly. Proof, right? But the "proof" of Albert Einstein's universe meant that Newton's idea of it didn't hold up anymore.

Back to the philosophy of science textbooks. They tell us we are supposed to get something extra once we have scientific proof. Newton predicted planetary movements, and Einstein predicted certain measurements to do with light. And they were both right, in context. Much of the magic of science comes from its apparent ability to predict future events or to understand unexamined cases because of its experience of examined ones.

The 18th-century Scottish philosopher David Hume threw a wrench into those works when he pointed out that science doesn't really ever absolutely prove *anything*. The famous example of this, first used much later by Karl Popper, about whom a little more to come, has to do with swans, of all things.

If for some reason you got interested in the color of swans, the scientific method would tell you to go out and have a look at some of them. So you get a folding chair and sit yourself on the bank of the Danube River and start watching. You see a white one, and another white one, and eventually lots of white ones. And the next day you go back again and see a hundred or more swans, all of them white. At this point the idea might form in your mind that swans are white, or even that *all* swans are white. And according to your limited experience so far, this idea would be correct. Then a black swan appears. The idea that all swans are white is, of course, destroyed.

"Scientific laws," which are built up from observations, are never 100 percent reliable. Hume pointed out that it doesn't make any difference how many white swans you see—there might always be a black one. There is no final certainty using the scientific method. If we're talking about predicting the future, the notion that all swans are white means that the next one coming around the corner on the river will be white. But will it?

Another philosopher, Karl Popper, put this a different way in the 1930s in Vienna, in his famous and still-current definition of what "scientific" means. He said that the central characteristic of a scientific belief is that it is *falsifiable*. Wait a minute. Isn't the big deal about science that it is *provable?* Not so, said Professor Popper. What is unscientific about astrology is that you can never prove it wrong. What is scientific about Einstein's theory of relativity is that if there were ever a reliable observation out of line with its predictions, the theory would be falsified. Gone into the historical garbage heap along with the conviction that the earth is flat.

I love that humility about a real scientific idea. "I'm only around as long as nobody proves me wrong," it says. And then it sits out in open view and waits for somebody to do just that. This is a humility not respected by health science practitioners, as we will see.

I hope you are starting to wonder about the authority of the so-called scientific material oozing out of your TV set. How much of it withstands the test of falsifiability? And how sure can we really be of science's predictions about the future?

The kind of science that the medical system relies on and that informs TV news stories involves probability and populations. It is called "epidemiology." In physics, a generalization (usually called a theory or a law) like Newton's description of gravity must apply in all cases or it's false. If it ever proved not to be predictive of future measurements confirming its truth, it's finished. Newton's and Einstein's physics meet Karl Popper's falsifiability.

Epidemiology dares make no such claims. On the contrary, its examination of probability in populations puts zero importance on the next observation—or on any observation. Its conclusions are trends. Epidemiology can tell us, for example, the proportion of male to female babies that will be born in a year, but it can't tell us whether the next baby will be a boy or girl. Any halfway competent insurance company epidemiologist will be bang on about the average date of death of the company's clients but will certainly be wrong about the date of death of every one of those clients.

Epidemiology in medicine is about people and is based on the assumption that people are similar. For example, we all have a liver, blood that circulates, a brain, weight never greater than thirteen hundred pounds. But trouble arises when we assume we all have similar characteristics that not everybody actually has—intact memory, ability to move around the environment effortlessly, liver and kidney function close to some norm, and willingness to behave according to certain rules, for example. An assumption of similarity is necessary for most science and works perfectly when you are dealing with electrons, molecules of potassium, or volumes of a pure gas such as helium. The more complicated the things being studied, the less similar they tend to be. Countries, banks, marriages, Labrador retrievers, and people are all potentially pretty complicated. Epidemiology is fine as long as it is talking about something that *is* the same for all individuals, whether they are Inuit, infant, disabled, demented, angry, vegetarian, or sick in the hospital. Otherwise, look out.

But epidemiology is the science, the only science, used to justify most medical treatment. Every day, millions of times over, we use its information about populations to decide the treatment of individuals. Is that okay? Epidemiology's predictions (about when someone will die, for example) are generalities. They are correct about the average but have nothing to say about any particular case. When we use epidemiology to predict someone's future, we are using quite reliable information about *absolutely nobody.*

The only way to falsify a conclusion reached by an epidemiology study would be to do another, somehow bigger or better or more convincing epidemiology study. So epidemiology is scientific in a way but fuzzy when it comes to falsifiability. Which actually makes it unscientific, according to the usual definition.

One of my patients illustrates this problem. Nellie Fedoruk is a survivor. At the age of seventy-eight she's had breast cancer and bowel cancer and operations for both of them. She's fine; the specialists lost interest in rechecking her years ago. Surgeons have also worked their magic on the blood vessels in her legs, the blood supply to her heart, and three of her four major weight-bearing joints. She's still walking around her little, perfectly maintained bungalow smoking cigarettes. Her husband, Arthur, died of a brain hemorrhage about a year and a half ago, and frankly, Nellie survived that, too, with flying colors. Her daughter, Michelle, is a busy insurance executive in a big city a thousand miles away, but she gets down to visit her mother four or five times a year.

I started seeing Nellie at home because problems with her legs kept her from easily getting out of the house. Her memory is fine, but she is incredibly fussy. The fussiness has a good side—her life is extremely orderly—but it does boil over into anxiety at times. And once in a while Nellie gets uptight enough to reach for her old friend rum and cola—too much rum and cola.

Nellie Fedoruk has diabetes and takes two types of pills for it. Her blood sugar is unpredictable and not often in the nice, safe textbook range where it should be. The problem is that Nellie gets in a tizzy and forgets to take her medication, so her blood sugar goes up. When she feels a little less anxious again, she remembers the medication and takes a little extra. If the tizzy is bad enough in the first place, she might have taken a few drinks in the evening, which also doesn't help her blood sugar or the chances of her taking her diabetes pills in any kind of reasonable way.

Then every couple of months Michelle flies into town, camps in the spare room for a few days, and straightens her mother's life out. This includes making sure Nellie takes every single one of her medications every single time she's supposed to. Michelle is a very orderly person; the acorn does not fall far from the tree.

Several times in the last year or two Nellie has fainted and landed in the hospital with low blood sugar. Sometimes this happens when Michelle is in town and makes Nellie take *all* her blood sugar-lowering medication, sometimes it happens when Nellie has been drinking, and sometimes it happens when she realizes she's missed her medication and decides she needs a double dose.

I face a real problem as her doctor. Seventy-eight is young by the standards of my practice, and Nellie could in theory live another dozen years or more. Some of the trouble diabetes can cause late in life might still be preventable by keeping her blood sugar closely and carefully controlled. But Nellie has gotten into serious practical problems every time I try to increase the dose of her diabetes medicine. Her life is just chaotic in a way that, in practical terms, nobody is going to be able to control.

I maintain Nellie on the very minimum amount of diabetes medicine that keeps her from getting into danger from really high blood sugar. Her diabetes blood test numbers are always awful by every textbook standard, but there is no other way to keep her from the more serious danger of *low* blood sugar.

Reenter epidemiology. Based on the experience of thousands of patients, it tells me that in general, diabetics won't get diabetes complications as soon if their diabetes is tightly controlled. That's if a close check is kept on their blood sugar and other measures of diabetic control and if the medication is adjusted as often as necessary to keep the blood sugar down. And if they are put on another preventive medication to protect the kidneys. That's the probability in that population. But probability and population are both abstract ideas that say nothing about the individual, real-life situation of Nellie Fedoruk.

Nassim Taleb is a probability mathematician who is also a stock-market trader. In his book *Fooled by Randomness,* he explains that probability can be characterized by how much randomness is associated with it. Probability with a lot of randomness is just what we get when we try to measure anything about fragile elderly people. And big-league, out-of-control randomness is anathema to generalities like the ones epidemiology produces about diabetes.

Nellie Fedoruk's future is not predicted by the epidemiology relevant to her disease, diabetes. She is atypical enough that the rules don't apply to her, for obvious practical reasons that anyone with common sense can see. And where the people in my practice are concerned, Nellie Fedoruk is typical. The difference between fragile elderly diabetics and younger diabetics is heterogeneity. The young ones tend to be similar with respect to all the things medicine measures. The fragile elderly tend to be very different. Typically atypical, you might say. They're all like that!

The example of Nellie may help you to understand how my medical practice has turned me into an agnostic. Epidemiology's generalizations about probability in populations are wrong so often in my practice that I have become very cautious—skeptical, in fact—about them. When I draw one conclusion from examining a group and exactly the opposite one from examining an individual, I need to be able to make a choice. Practicing medicine the way I do, for the people who are my patients, I have absolutely no question in my mind about that choice.

I can hear good friends and colleagues—a hard-core epidemiologist, evidence-based internal-medicine specialist, or endocrinologist, for example—saying, "Of course the rules apply to Mrs. Fedoruk. It's just that she's not taking her medication properly and she drinks." I'm sorry; this kind of thinking is seriously, dangerously backwards. My responsibility, and ours in medicine, is to the patients. When we start thinking that we are first responsible for providing consistent rules, and then the people need to conform to those, and that when they don't that's just too bad, then we really quit doing what we're paid for and begin to do harm. As I think of my dear friends whose practice and philosophy are evidence based, I know perfectly well that each of them has the best interests of their patients at heart, too. But that's not what we're teaching students and not what we present as the best we have to offer.

When scientific rules of medical practice derived from epi-demiology say one thing and common sense about the seventy-eight-year-old lady in front of me this afternoon says something completely different, I have no trouble making that choice. *She's* real. Epidemiology's predictions about her future are not. Attractive though abstractions are, they can never replace our real-world responsibility to other people.

Epidemiology's most important tool is the randomized con-trolled trial. When health professionals, journalists, and mem-bers of the public talk about scientific evidence in health care, this tool is what everybody is talking about. These trials are, in our ordinary language, scientific experiments. They can be very simple, but they are usually incredibly complicated.

The whole collected group of randomized controlled trials on any question in medicine is called the "evidence base." This evidence base may, depending on whom you talk to, include all the studies that have ever been done on the subject, only the studies that have been published, only the studies that were con-trolled, only the studies that have end points that seem to make sense, only the studies not funded by drug industry, and so on.

Randomized controlled trials typically involve hundreds or thousands of subjects (people), millions of dollars, big organiza-tions such as drug companies or government research agencies, and years of organization and work. There is a billion-dollar in-dustry of research design consultants, research-conducting or-ganizations, statistical analysts, ethics review boards, and the journals that assist in the production and publication of these studies.

The reliability of these huge and influential experiments is rarely questioned. But we can already figure out that they suf-fer from the weaknesses of their mother science, epidemiology.

The results tell us, at best, what probabilities are in populations. Theoretical and approximate. They matter to each of us only if we really are members of the artificial populations set up for the trials. If not, in no way does the outcome of any trial predict *our* particular future. Quite a few approximations for a science that we depend on for the rules of medical care, don't you think?

Especially if we happen to be unusual. Like pretty well every single one of my patients. Randomized controlled trials tell us about a group of people given a treatment (usually a drug treatment) compared with a similar group given no treatment. Are any of the "subjects" in the trial anything like Elizabeth O'Malley or Nellie Fedoruk?

Is the question the trial is trying to answer meaningful to these people (would it matter, for example, to Elizabeth O'Malley if her bone density changed by 1 or 2 percent)? More generally, could there be a bias to a clinical trial's outcome because the doctors doing the trials are paid by drug industry sponsors or because their careers are advanced by a positive result or because the drug company doing the trial benefits from a positive result? Does it matter that trials that show that a drug works are more likely to be published? Are we concerned because once there are several positive randomized controlled trials for a particular treatment, it becomes unethical to test it any further?

Ironically, very important rules of ethics can weaken the logical relevance of trials that use them. For sound ethical reasons, frail elderly people are excluded from drug trials, and often the necessary confirming trials simply aren't allowed.

Clinical trials are the best method we have come up with so far for "proving" the benefit of a treatment. A chain is as strong as its weakest link. And the randomized controlled trial as it is practiced and interpreted in today's medical system involves a very long chain and quite a few corroded links. That chain starts with an idea (commercial, scientific, career oriented, or however it gets into someone's mind), and it ends when Elizabeth O'Malley or Mary McCarthy gets out of the hospital on a ton of preventive drugs.

Why did randomized controlled trials assume such overwhelming importance? The answer is that reliability and consistency appear to be assured by its methods. And reliability and consistency are important for several reasons.

Business, insurers, government health care agencies, and policy makers all need reliability. More reliable care should mean a better outcome for a population, but we only get that if the health care rules that epidemiology coughs up for us are applied consistently. And the more consistency we accomplish, the less likely we are to accommodate the needs of outliers—oddballs. People who could never have been members of the original study population, who don't fit the mold.

Clinical guidelines are supposed to give us consistency. These are like recipes for health care (which is why I call their consistent use "cookbook care"). Clinical guidelines are evidence based: they come from the information gathered from randomized controlled trials. These days there are several different guidelines for most common clinical problems. This happens because different experts have different opinions about what trials should be included in the evidence base. But the tendency is not toward diversity among the guidelines.

I have been teaching medical students and residents in family practice for decades; it is one of the most enjoyable and stimulating parts of a full practice. Without trying to criticize any of the lovely people who have put up with my quirky teaching style, I have noticed a trend over the years that I think comes from the guidelines approach to care. Students trained recently are very likely to recommend identical treatment—identical to what their classmates would recommend and identical for every patient. This trend isn't confined to medical students. Nutritionists, pharmacists, and other health care professionals coming out of their training programs also tend to be consistent in their proposed treatment.

This is no surprise. If we wanted to get the best possible benefit for the largest number of people, and if we believed that randomized controlled trials give us really reliable information about benefits, we would do our best to pull together the results of those trials and write down the best treatment, creating clinical guidelines. There's not much point in doing this unless we make sure the people giving the treatment always give that same best treatment. And what better place to start than the schools where we train the professionals?

What I'm seeing among my students is the result—consistency. The evidence-based, guidelines-driven approach is working like a charm. I try as hard as I can to get these wonderful students to *think*: is this treatment really safe and helpful for this old man we're seeing? Sometimes it's an uphill battle, and not because these young students aren't smart enough.

This situation worries me because at the same time as we are teaching young doctors, pharmacists, and nurses to practice according to reliable evidence, we might be discouraging them from thinking creatively about unusual one-off situations. Over my few decades of practice I've seen an evolution in the culture of health care professionals. Consistency has replaced preparation for the unexpected; answers have replaced questions. The state of the art is the state of the science. Not, as far as I can tell, necessarily a good thing.

Consistency is self-reinforcing. As clinical guidelines for common diseases become better defined, there is less and less chance that experts will disagree with one another about the most effective treatment. There is a certain machinery in the way we do business that guarantees this kind of pulling together of opinion.

Imagine for a moment that a doctor, under pressure, tired, and driven nuts by a really bad day full of ungrateful people who blame him for problems he didn't cause and can't do anything about, doesn't get along with someone whose family member gets sicker and dies, in spite of treatment. Imagine that the doctor looked at the guidelines for treatment and realized they couldn't possibly apply to this person and decided not to follow them. He treated the *person,* not the population, as his best instinct and common sense told him he should. And then he failed to show grace under pressure when the son was looking for someone to blame for his mother's misfortune.

It is well known that people who sue doctors and other health professionals do it not because they didn't get better but because things went badly and the doctor acted as if he were infallible and failed to communicate. If there is a malpractice lawsuit, the outcome will depend on the testimony of experts, who will say that clinical guidelines should have been followed. It takes a creative and determined ordinary general practitioner to run that kind of risk, to break the rules, even when the rules don't make sense.

Recently there have been some changes to the way doctors are paid where I work. Some of these are wonderful from my point of view. The house-call fee item was increased. Nursing home care is now better paid, and there is a lot more money for each service for the very elderly. All good. But payment bonuses also exist for following clinical guidelines. This sword cuts both ways. Just as we are paid to be consistent, we are paid to be rigid. One size fits all.

Clinical guidelines kick in for every doctor when a patient meets a disease definition. More and more these days, diseases (or being at risk) are defined to make care consistent and to avoid dependence on "soft" clinical findings like a complaint of pain, swelling of a joint, or sounds the doctor hears through a stethoscope. Blood tests and results of measurements by machines are reassuringly black-and-white when it comes to whether you have the disease or not and whether or not you are treated according to guidelines. The disease definitions are often written directly into the guidelines so that there can be no mistake.

Diabetes is defined strictly by a blood test. I went to a local laboratory early one morning because I woke up with an irregular heartbeat and wanted to confirm what it was with a cardiogram. At the same time, I got a bunch of "routine" blood tests done to send to my family doctor. My fasting blood glucose was 6.1; diabetic by just a hair. I was very relieved when a repeat test was just below the definition of the disease. My doctor, always reassuring and of course never wrong, told me that it was the stress of the irregular heartbeat that had put my blood sugar up. I was happy to agree.

Heart attack is now diagnosed by a blood test. Heart failure, which is a different thing, to do with the heart's function, is also now defined by a measurement tool outside the hands of the examining doctor: an echocardiogram. Osteoporosis is defined by a bone-density reading from a machine. Elevated cholesterol is defined by a blood test, and so on. It's almost as if you didn't need the doctor to make the diagnosis. There is very little room even

for the interpretation of the diagnosis, and because the guidelines are usually pretty clear, you probably also don't need the
doctor to tell you what the treatment is going to be.

This is part of the whole movement toward reliability, consistency, and reproducibility in diagnosis and treatment. Not only
do we define the treatment in clear, consistent, absolute terms,
we also define the disease that way. No human error: you have it
or you don't.

And I can see my doctor friends shaking their heads. What is
he worried about? Does he want us to go back to the days when
diabetes was defined as passing huge amounts of urine and being always thirsty? Should we wait for someone to show up in
the emergency room gasping for breath before we diagnose
heart failure? Please. The sword has two edges. Of course we
gain when consistency leads to earlier diagnosis and more ac-
curate treatment. I'm simply saying what we all know already:
the price we pay for greater consistency is a less flexible attitude
toward treating outliers. And the fragile elderly are nearly all
outliers.

The medical system is wonderful as long as you can benefit
from what it has to offer. It is scientific but involves a kind of
science loaded with questionable assumptions, such as the idea
that everybody is similar, and partly sound logic, such as ex-
tending conclusions from one group to a different one. Many of
its assumptions are conditional: you're going to be fine as long
as you resemble everybody else. Scientific studies have moved
to the center of the medical universe, and everything is considered legitimate to the extent that it aligns with the studies' methods and results. We are out to prevent death and disease and,
when we can't, to rescue people from them. Consistency in care

is guaranteed because scientific evidence informs clinical guide-lines that everyone follows.

Is it possible to be scientific about doing medical care with-out having to live with and follow the rules of the kind of science that powers epidemiology and clinical guidelines? What about a scientific study, a clinical trial, where the size of the population is *one*? Is there a crisis response that would work better for certain people than dialing 911? Would anyone even want to think about such things?

# 3 Poisonous Prevention
## Just Keep Takin' Them Pills

**DICK HALSTADT**

Dr. Halstadt was one of the most stubborn people I had ever met. He was a retired internal medicine specialist and spent his middle years practicing in a hospital. He had also had a reputation as a high-speed daredevil. He drove the fastest car, and his boat held speed records; he had survived some newsworthy accidents and also did his share of carousing, including disappearing for several days at a time, driving his poor wife to distraction.

The doctor had suffered some financial reverses in later years after his wife died of cancer. When I picked him up as a patient, he was a lot slower moving and lived in a small apartment. He confided that he didn't have much money left. Our story opens on a roasting-hot summer day, with me in shorts and sandals banging on his door. I was finally let in to find Dr. Halstadt sweating and red faced, with the television going full blast and the temperature in the room close to one hundred degrees Fahrenheit. After checking him over, asking him to reduce the dose of his blood pressure medication, and telling him for God's sake to open some windows, drink some Gatorade, and get himself downstairs into the yard where there was some shade, I arranged to come back and see him in another week.

During that week, his son took him in to see a specialist, the next-generation internist in Dr. Halstadt's old practice. A couple of weeks later I got a letter from this doctor telling me that the old man was in heart failure and that the doctor had added three medications to prevent the problem from getting worse, including a water pill (diuretic). On my next visit, the temperature in the apartment was still unbearably hot, and my patient was staggering around and confused. I looked in the fridge: nothing but rotten food. Had he been spending the afternoon downstairs in the shade? "Bugger that. No TV down there." The windows were shut.

The signs of dehydration were unmistakable, and Dr. Halstadt's blood pressure was very low. I told him I thought he might need to go to emergency to get rehydrated. "Piss off," was the response. I asked him to stop the water pill and punched them out of his blister pack. Although water pills treat heart failure, they have the dangerous side effect of dehydration, especially when someone is perspiring and not drinking enough. I called the son and left a strongly worded message on his answering machine that his dad needed to get outside in the afternoon and drink plenty of liquid. I scheduled to see Dr. Halstadt in two days.

My next contact was a call from a medical student at the hospital. Dr. Halstadt had fallen at home. He was not injured but was dehydrated. He had been taking the water pill in full doses (he must've retrieved them from the garbage).

He tolerated rehydration, got back on his feet, and then discharged himself from the hospital against medical advice, calling a cab and returning to his apartment wearing pajamas and a dressing gown. Luckily, the weather cooled off, Dr. Halstadt stopped taking the water pill (because a heart specialist in the hospital had told him it wasn't necessary), and life went on. He continued to feel dizzy and to run a low blood pressure because of his preventive heart failure medicine, but he absolutely refused to make any changes.

### DAVID SCARLATTI

I'll never forget the first time I saw Dave. The family had called me to see if I could do something about his chest pain, and even I, who imagine I've seen every kind of home living situation, was stunned by the condition of his house. It was a terribly run-down place facing a big, busy street. Getting to the front door involved stepping carefully on the very edge of the wooden stairway because half the boards were rotted through. The front door, made of plywood, was hard to knock on because the outer layer was wavy from years of blowing rain. Inside—wow! The odor was so complicated I had trouble separating urine from cat from rotten food from wet basement. Curling linoleum from the 1940s, a gas stove black with decades of dribbled food, and filthy, shiny, sticky furniture completed the decor. "Original," a good realtor would call it.

Dave was not a happy man. He just moaned and stared around the room in obvious distress, grasped at the front of his shirt, and never gave any coherent answers to questions. His daughter Carlene, who chain-smoked, said she wasn't sure how long he had been this way, but she was certain there was no way in hell he was leaving the house. No hospital, no doctor's office, no tests, nothing. He had always been terrified of these things, and she intended to respect that, she said, thoughtfully blowing blue smoke sideways away from my face.

After several weeks of trial and error I had figured out (1) Dave was very demented, (2) he was somehow surviving on prepared food that Carlene brought each week and stored in the fridge, (3) he had no chest pain (or much of anything else physically the matter that I could find), and (4) most of his distress and terror had to do with his usual (lifelong, it seemed) response to anything new or different. He was just that kind of guy. We carried on on that basis, and I visited him every few weeks, always on the day Carlene was there.

Several months later something went wrong. Over a couple of weeks, Dave wasn't dressing himself or even getting out of bed. I had to see him upstairs in his bedroom, which involved a whole new aesthetic experience I had been hoping to avoid. When I examined him, his blood pressure was a little low, but I couldn't find any real reason for his sudden change in function. I did tests (the laboratory came in and drew blood) and examined him again and again, but his sudden new immobility was still a mystery. Carlene started talking about a nursing home.

On my way out the door a week or so later, she took me aside and told me that her sister from California had been in town for a month, and Carlene had just found out that the sister, horrified at Dave's distress, had taken him out in her car to a heart specialist to see about his chest pain. How she accomplished this I have no idea. Carlene also discovered that the sister had a blister pack of five or six medications that the heart specialist had prescribed and was coming in and giving them to Dave every morning.

When I phoned the cardiologist, she explained that Dave had angina and was now on proper treatment to prevent a heart attack. Once the sister left town, we slowly stopped the drugs, and Dave went back to business as usual.

Dave Scarlatti had preventable heart disease like my '84 diesel car has preventable heart disease.

I'VE DESCRIBED THE fragile elderly, a group of people I'm very familiar with. I've also outlined the characteristics of the medical system I work in. The two are incompatible because the medical system is hell-bent on rescue and prevention, and the result for the elderly people in my practice tends to be too much medication and horrifying, expensive, futile, and sometimes fatal trips to the hospital. In this chapter I take a look at the first of these problems: prevention.

To question the idea that an ounce of prevention is worth a pound of cure seems ridiculous. And this idea has led to a medical system focused on prevention, which is more and more about rules and less and less about common sense or judgment based on the relationship between a person trained to give health care and somebody who is receiving it. We call these rules "best practice." For my patients, they rarely are.

Here's an example of how best-practice health care works for the general population—people other than the fragile elderly. When I was practicing in a city family practice office, a fellow I'll call Darren visited me regularly. Darren was a forty-year-old management consultant and a textbook conventional-health-risk train wreck. He smoked. He ate everything in sight, especially high-trans-fat stuff like frozen strawberry pies, Twinkies, and convenience-store pepperoni, so he was sixty pounds overweight. His blood pressure was high, his cholesterol and blood sugar likewise. We always had the same conversation, in which I would look at all the numbers (which were awful no matter how much medication I gave him) and tell Darren he had to straighten things out or he was headed for trouble. Sweaty and nervous and in an even bigger hurry than I was, Darren always sang the same song: "I'm two weeks away from the end of this project. As soon as it's done, I'll have tons of time with no travel, no late nights, no pressure, time with the kids, a chance to exercise, and a *much* better diet." But Darren's projects tended to overlap.

Well, Darren had a rare happy ending. He got away on holiday with his wife, went to a meditation-based facility in Arizona, came back with a whole new outlook, changed jobs, quit smoking, lost weight. He turned out still to need some blood pressure and cholesterol medication to keep his numbers within international guidelines, but he took his pills, and we were both a lot happier.

Thing is, Darren, as part of his holiday conversion experience, finally understood that he was a member of a high-risk group. He realized that he had better follow the rules for treatment that I offered him. For high blood pressure it would be lifestyle advice and eventually some medication. Both Darren and I were making a prediction about an outcome as part of the contract between us.

My prescription for his problems came straight from the best-practice rules. If the patient understands the instructions, reduces salt in his food, takes the medication as prescribed, and comes back in two weeks, chances are his blood pressure will be better. And much more important, better blood pressure predicts a better health outcome. No stroke, or at least a delayed stroke.

Modern preventive health care is a tidy, predictable, uniform, reproducible package. And its aim is reasonable and quite straightforward: prevent the disaster before it happens. Who could argue with that?

Real, sensible prevention provides definite benefits. If the targeted population is the same as the population in studies of the preventive treatment, if the studies are convincing, if they're properly done and properly interpreted, if the cost is reasonable, if the treatment is safe, and if the benefit is real, none of us would fail to practice prevention. You'll notice there are six "ifs."

An example is taking aspirin to thin the blood to prevent a stroke when you have a heart rhythm disturbance called atrial fibrillation. This one is close to home for me. About a year ago I had an episode of atrial fibrillation, which fortunately hasn't returned. But if it does, and if the rest of my health is good, I will start taking aspirin, since I'm similar to most of the people who have been in studies of the effect of taking aspirin on having a stroke when there is a rhythm disturbance. The chance of having a stroke in atrial fibrillation when you're taking aspirin is only a little lower, but it really is lower. The studies are convincing on this question, and many of them are very well done indeed. Aspirin is cheap, and though it has some side effects, rarely serious, they don't compare with the consequences of a stroke. And the benefit certainly is real. All the "ifs" are covered.

I don't doubt that preventive drugs can coincide with lower cholesterol, increased bone density, lower blood pressure, controlled blood sugar, and also fewer or later heart attacks, strokes, or fractures and even longer life. But this basket of benefits is likely real only for the kind of people involved in the studies that showed those benefits. Most of the time they were people who had nothing else the matter with them. For the fragile elderly those benefits are questionable and pretty well unprovable even if they exist. But medical practice guidelines don't normally warn us about these limitations. And the result is some of the problems I've already discussed.

There are two problems with prevention as we practice it, when applied to fragile elderly people. First, it suffers from some apparently overwhelming logical absurdities. Second, even if it worked in these people, is it really what we want to accomplish? Taking medication every day to increase bone density to prevent a fracture is an example. The changes in bone density are tiny, changes in fracture rates are also very small, and any change at all takes a long time—longer than many fragile elderly people will live. Are the results really worth the trouble fragile elderly people go to to get them? I don't think so.

Yet we continue with prevention even when it no longer makes any sense. Part of the reason is that we don't know when and where to stop. Medical science doesn't give doctors a sharp line (or any line, really) between people who should be getting the full preventive treatment and others who shouldn't. Many doctors, therefore, don't draw the line at all. Everybody gets cookbook care from the cradle to the grave. One size fits all. But when it comes to clinical science's guidelines or rules, fragile elderly people are black swans, of the kind I talked about describing limitations of and exceptions to scientific laws. Bad things can happen when, as we have heard said in a different but oddly related context, you're black in a white world.

Isn't it true that if we fasten seatbelts, we are likelier to survive a crash? Nobody would question washing your hands in a hospital. Taking your malaria drugs before going to Africa is reasonable based on common sense, right?

Right. But there are two kinds of prevention: the kind that makes sense, like common sense, and the other kind. Recklessness where health and safety are concerned is dangerous and should be discouraged, but if I do up my seatbelt and take my malaria drugs, does that really *cause* a difference in what happens in an accident and whether I get sick going to Africa? And what if somebody (whom I was convinced had an inside track of knowledge) told me that walking around the house four times in the morning before heading off to work would increase my productivity? Would I still do it even though it didn't seem to make a lot of sense?

Epidemiologists tell us that one of the most important factors supporting *cause*, when two sets of events seem related, is a commonsense explanation for *why* they would be related. It's the difference between "I fell against the mirror, it broke, and it caused me to cut myself" and "I fell against the mirror, it broke, and it caused me to have seven years of bad luck." The first cause statement is reasonable according to common sense, and the second not so much.

The truth is that there often isn't a commonsense explanation for why taking a particular medication is believed to lead to prevention of a particular disease, or event, in the future. Sometimes there is a fanciful explanation, understandable in some way to experts in a particular area of medical research and based on ideas about biology that may or may not exist in the real world. Most of us, even doctors, can't recognize the direct, reasonable, sensible machinery behind many of those explanations for prevention. Very often all you can be sure exists is a coincidence, *probably* not due to chance alone, between some action and some result, in a drug trial. I call prevention based on coincidence of this kind, where there is no commonsense reason for the coincidence, "noncommonsense" prevention.

I'm told, for example, that if I take my cholesterol drugs, the amount of cholesterol in my blood will decrease. Cholesterol builds up on the inside of arteries and eventually blocks them, presumably causing heart attacks and strokes. Anything that keeps the amount of cholesterol in the blood down will at least slow down that dangerous buildup inside my arteries. Simple explanation, and approximately what lives in most people's minds when they think about cholesterol and heart disease.

But nobody has seen this sequence actually happening. We can't directly observe blobs of cholesterol attaching themselves to the insides of arteries, and we also can't see a change in that process that results from less cholesterol in the bloodstream. What we are shown are animated cartoons of these events, played to us over and over again to help us understand why we should take our cholesterol medication and stop eating fat. The process is inferred—presumed—based on things we can measure. That piling up of little bits of cholesterol inside the arteries makes a sort of sense we can imagine and becomes something we believe in when we watch the cartoon. But the relationship of blood cholesterol to heart attacks and strokes is much, much more complicated. And nobody—*nobody*—understands it completely.

Still, people with an enthusiasm for our taking cholesterol drugs, through whatever motivation—humanitarian, financial, or ambiguous—construct simplistic cartoons to help us understand. The commonsense explanation is not out there in front of our faces, like the reason we keep three-year-olds off busy streets. It is produced for us fancifully because the real explanation is too complicated, hasn't yet been discovered, or doesn't exist.

Recently a doctor who does TV commentary on health care described a study in which people who lived close to their relatives were less likely to be depressed (never mind, depending on your relatives, whether you might think it should be the opposite!). The doctor didn't have to state the conclusion that viewers were expected to reach: keeping your relatives close will prevent you from getting depressed. That conclusion is just assumed from the correlation between being unhappy and having your relatives a long way away. But what if generally crabby, hard-to-get-along-with people tend both to stay away from their family and to get depressed? Then the cause-and-effect, potentially preventive conclusion would be a little different. And, to go a step further, what if it were true that moving most potentially depressed people closer to their relatives made them less likely to get depressed, and so some well-meaning effort is made to move an exceptionally crabby, hard-to-get-along-with person next door to his brother and things work in reverse: they fight and end up in trouble. Why then would this type of prevention, not based on a commonsense or a scientifically sound reason, be practiced?

Imagine a doctor gives you something for your nausea. You know right away whether the treatment makes you stop throwing up or not. But if the doctor gives you something to prevent some event in the future, usually because you have a risk factor like high blood pressure or high cholesterol, the only reason you would take the medicine every day is that it has been shown in reliable trials to do what it is supposed to—to prevent you from having trouble in the future, to predict your future and change it. You don't feel any better, you don't feel any worse, and, a bit frightening for some people, you can never really know whether the drug worked in your individual case. You have your heart attack now, in five years, or never.

What would have happened if you hadn't taken the preventive drug? Nobody ever knows what would have happened.

The reason nobody knows is that "what would have happened" doesn't exist. Epidemiological information is about no particular thing. About nothing, from the point of view of your particular circumstance.

The justification for preventive drugs, where there is no commonsense explanation for their preventive effect, comes from drug trials alone, which are supposed to predict the benefit. And now that we've struggled through understanding the randomized controlled trial and some of its problems, we may not feel as secure in relying on drug trials as justification for prevention, as we originally did when the TV journalist, family doctor, or international expert told us we should take a particular medication to prevent us from getting sick. All the more so if we are unusual in many ways, like most fragile elderly people.

There is another theoretical worry about prevention. This has to do with Karl Popper's definition of "scientific." Are these medical studies falsifiable? Well, yes and no. You could show that a trial of prevention leads to a false conclusion, but only by doing some bigger or otherwise more credible trial. None of the individual results in a trial of prevention amounts to proof or disproof of anything.

If I take my cholesterol-lowering medication, exercise every day, eat healthfully, get my blood pressure checked regularly, and then have a heart attack at age fifty, it doesn't falsify anything. My outcome, and the early heart attacks of who knows how many other people, are considered *exceptions*. When the future predicted by epidemiology doesn't come true for me, the explanation is that the statement about prevention in the population was never about *me*. The generality of population-based information means that it does not meet the usually accepted definition of "scientific." There can be any number of contrary events, but the prediction is still not subject to true science's safety valve of falsifiability.

But isn't it me (or you, or your mother, or anybody else) who matters when we try to do "medical care"? As a philosopher friend of mine said once, "I'd much rather be a member of a group that has a 10 percent chance of a free trip to Hawaii than a group that has a 5 percent chance." So would I. And this statement applies to prevention of the noncommonsense type, as long as the group we're talking about exists and we really are members of it. Each of us either gets a free trip or not. But whether we do or not, it's pretty hard to be sure which "group" we were in, or whether the groups even exist at all, unless we completely credit the people who are offering the trips to Hawaii, believe completely in the reliability of the machinery of the lottery, and don't have some strange disqualifying characteristics that make it very unlikely we are a member of any group at all.

Studies that show that a drug, for example, is associated with a good outcome, where no commonsense connection exists between the drug and the outcome, create imaginary groups of people: the ones who take the drug and the ones who don't. But in the real world, the groups are made up of people who may be very different from those who are hoping for benefit.

Prevention today usually means prevention using medication. But there are three reasons beyond these theoretical ones to be very skeptical about preventive medication in fragile elderly people. I call these the three logical absurdities of prevention in the elderly.

The first logical absurdity is that no frail or fragile elderly person is ever included in any preventive drug trial. We know very well that the guidelines for treating disease risk states (high blood pressure, high cholesterol, and low bone density, for example) are evidence based, which means they are built up from the results of randomized controlled trials. Those trials are done using volunteers, and those volunteers are quite carefully screened. There are two very interesting double-edged swords in the ethics of doing randomized controlled trials that guarantee that the fragile elderly are excluded.

Sword one: even in randomized controlled trials where the word "elderly" appears in the title, the rules followed by the ethics review boards who must approve every trial exclude an awful lot of people. This is as it should be. Bringing people into an experiment where they get given drugs is potentially dangerous. One way to limit that danger is not to let anyone participate who looks likely to get into trouble. So when we read the exclusion criteria for absolutely every randomized controlled trial done these days, we see that nobody with anything wrong with them (except the disease being studied in the trial) is ever included. You're diabetic? Sorry. Take pain medication for arthritis? Next! Smoke cigarettes, have a history of depression, liver function not perfect, taking any medication? No participation for you.

This would be why we never see preventive drug trials involving people like my elderly patients: nearly all of them have exclusion criteria, because they have lots of illnesses. So a researcher would have a terrible time finding enough, say, ninety-year-olds who could ethically be run through her drug trial. And even if, combing the whole population of a country like the United States, somebody *did* come up with the two or three hundred completely healthy ninety-year-olds needed to see whether, for example, lowering blood pressure prevents strokes in that age group, she'd be studying an extremely unusual bunch of ninety-year-olds, not representatives of that age group at all.

Most people involved with health care of the elderly are aware of the HYVET (hypertension in the very elderly trial), an ongoing study of treatment of high blood pressure in people eighty years of age or older. The stated rationale is to settle the issue of whether very elderly people should be treated for high blood pressure, since nearly all previous trials limited the age of participants. The published report of this trial in the prestigious *New England Journal of Medicine* in 2008 does not include the full list of exclusion criteria but states that they

> include a contraindication to the use of the trial medications, accelerated hypertension, secondary hypertension, hemorrhagic stroke in the previous six months, heart failure requiring treatment with antihypertensive medication, a serum creatinine level greater than 150 μmol per liter, a serum potassium level of less than 3.5 mmol per liter or more than 5.5 mmol per liter, gout, a diagnosis of clinical dementia, and the requirement of nursing care.

There are other exclusion criteria that aren't mentioned. The HYVET trial shows reduction in deaths from all causes and reduction in strokes with the treatment. Far from settling the question of whether to treat the fragile elderly for high blood pressure, however, this trial just confirms the fundamental inability of trials of this kind ever to address the question properly. The people in it are very elderly, but they are not remotely fragile.

The second double-edged ethical sword is that ethics watchdogs—perfectly correctly—insist that anybody who gets to be in a drug trial (or, for that matter, any experiment designed to test the effect of anything on health) knows exactly what he's getting into. This is called informed consent. Now at times—studying treatment for dementia, for example—guardians or "authorized representatives" are allowed to consent on behalf of incompetent people. But to be included in nearly any study, you have to be able to understand a quite long and involved consent form. This would eliminate about half of my patients, who can't understand or remember an awful lot of anything.

As logic loopholes go, not including fragile elderly in any trials looks like the kind you could drive a truck through. You would think that this would result in our being worried about whether fragile elderly people actually benefit from prevention with drugs. It doesn't take a person with a PhD in statistics to see the problem for what it is: you can't obtain evidence-based health information using randomized controlled trials unless you keep real-world elderly people with complicated problems away. To put this another way, it's impossible, using currently accepted procedure, to get evidence-based health information about the frail elderly, *period*. The result is that all my patients, and every similar elderly person, live in a kind of evidence-free zone.

As I've said, one defining characteristic of the fragile elderly is heterogeneity. They are all different from one another. This trait results in unpredictability. And in particular, their response to medication is unpredictable.

We understand there is medication that controls a symptom—that makes you feel better—and then there is medication that prevents a problem in the future. It's also clear that prevention based on clinical trials alone (the noncommonsense type of prevention) can be distinguished from prevention that is based on common sense, like taking an umbrella when it looks as though it might rain.

Prevention for you involves a prediction about *your* future. There is no reason to take a preventive treatment unless you believe you're going to have the same kind of response to it that the people in the randomized controlled trial showing its effect did (allegedly, probably, on average). No reason unless you believe that the evidence supporting the medicine is predictive about *your* future. But fragile elderly people's response to medication isn't predictable. How reasonable is it to give a treatment relying on a predictable response to somebody whose response isn't predictable? This is the second absurdity of prevention in these elderly people.

As discussed earlier, reporters, just trying to provide us with information we seem to want, troll the media releases from the prestigious health journals. One of the most common misinterpretations passed along to us by journalists is confusion about risk. An example will illustrate.

Say the next time you booked a flight across the country, you were offered a ticket on a plane with equipment that cut the chance of a crash in half. The special ticket on this better-equipped plane costs twice as much as the same flight on the ordinary old Boeing 737 you're used to. Do you buy the expensive, safer plane trip?

Of course not. But, insists the airline Web site, *you're cutting your risk by 50 percent!* How can you be so irresponsible? Don't you care about safety? Now you understand by intuition that there isn't really any value to cutting the risk of dying in a plane crash, however hideous, real, and quite possible that event might be. You're not ready to shell out an extra $500 to drop your risk from one in 11 million to one in 22 million. The risk is already acceptably low (and the flight already unacceptably expensive).

Statisticians refer to this difference as relative risk versus absolute risk. My risk of having a heart attack in the next twelve months can be calculated at about 1 percent. (Don't even ask.

The statistical categories boggle the mind. Just google "heart attack risk" for yourself and see if you can make any sense of it.) Reducing that by 50 percent of *relative risk* would appear on the surface to be an incredible benefit, worth going to almost any lengths to enjoy. But the absolute risk only drops by one half of one percent. Not quite so impressive. Would I take a drug every day for that? Quit smoking (I don't smoke)? Destroy my pleasure in eating?

The HYVET trial, by the way, reports its results of treating high blood pressure as "reduced total mortality by 21 percent and stroke mortality by 39 percent." Impressive. But plenty of people in the treated group also had strokes and died. The absolute risk reduction, a tiny fraction of these numbers, isn't mentioned. And I think you have to wonder why not.

For elderly people the price paid, even if prevention actually worked for them (which it doesn't), is usually far too high for the tiny increment of benefit they would receive. Not just the price in dollars, but the price in inconvenience, confusion, "medicalization" of their lives, and, of course, side effects.

When we talk about cutting risk for fragile elderly people by giving them medication, for example, it also matters *how long* it takes for that risk to be reduced. One of the characteristics of the fragile elderly is that they are near the end of their lives. How useful is it to take a medication every day, go on vitamins, or even eat food you hate if the imaginary health benefit (or even some real one) will take longer to land on your shoulders than you're likely to be around? Add this to the usual tiny change in absolute risk of preventive treatments, and we have the third absurdity of prevention in the fragile elderly. Even if the benefits exist, they are usually so minute that they would be nowhere near worth bothering with.

Not everyone agrees with this point of view. A medical friend of mine says he can't justify "cutting off" people from preventive benefit just because they're old. When I suggested that the particular lady we were talking about wasn't interested in preventing anything if it meant taking medication she hated, the doctor dismissively waved his hand in the air and said that that lady was an anecdote (just one individual) and that it's evidence that comes from big populations that counts. At this point I found I had to sit down.

Older people shouldn't be given preventive treatments they can't benefit from. But guidelines-based prescribing for old people is on the rise, not decreasing. Here's how this works in practice.

Fragile old people tend to have lots of illnesses, which include quite a long list of conditions that amount to "risk states," not really being *sick*, as our usual idea of illness might suggest. High cholesterol, high blood pressure, low bone density (osteoporosis), high blood sugar (diabetes), and low heart-pump function (congestive heart failure) are examples of these risk states. I've put them in that order on purpose. The ones at the beginning are pure risk states; just about nobody feels sick or suffers any loss of function from high blood pressure or high cholesterol themselves. At the end of the list are a couple of others you certainly can get sick and feel pretty awful with, even die from: diabetes and heart failure. But even diabetes and heart failure now exist in forms that don't make anybody feel ill. In their mildest form they are defined by blood tests and ultrasound. Unless you took the tests, you'd never know you had these "illnesses."

Every one of these conditions is diagnosed and properly treated by informed doctors according to a clinical guideline. The clinical guideline for treatment of each of these conditions involves drugs. If one medicine doesn't work, the guidelines typically advise adding a second one. And possibly a third. But an average person I would see at home because of advanced age and dependency doesn't just have one or two of these risk states; she has several. If you apply guideline diagnostic criteria, especially to a patient under stress such as an eighty-seven-year-old would experience in a typical emergency room scene, many of the fragile elderly would trip nearly all the diagnostic switches.

That tripping is, in a simple way, what happened to Dave Scarlatti in the cardiologist's office. It is also what happened in a much more comprehensive way to Mary McCarthy. And it happens thousands of times every day of every year in emergency rooms, family doctors' and specialists' offices, and hospitals all over the world. The consequences are variable, or heterogeneous. But they're never good. This is because benefit from this kind of preventive medication in this population logically doesn't exist. Even when there is no harm at all, the best outcome is that somebody feels the same as before, choking down handfuls of expensive drugs every day. What's called the cost-benefit ratio is never positive, because there is no benefit.

But it's not just about the money we waste giving useless medicines to people who can't benefit from them. It's the *harm* such patients face from being on too many drugs, and the wrong drugs. Another defining characteristic of that elderly patient population is that illnesses don't look the way the textbook says they should. Well, neither do drug side effects. In the same way that a ninety-year-old woman with appendicitis may just stop getting out of bed in the morning, when she gets the wrong drug she doesn't necessarily pop up with the rash, headache, or nausea that the drug package insert lists as usual side effects. She just "goes off." And for many old people, "going off" is a regular event.

You can also recognize this nonspecific reaction to medication in David Scarlatti's situation. The real risk of drugs in these people is immense and complicated but also obscure. Sudden loss of ability for someone like David Scarlatti can be caused by just about anything. But it's usually *something,* and as we say in primary care, common things are common. When a frail old person suddenly loses mobility, the cause is probably one from a not-too-long list. A friend of mine who is also a wonderful geriatric doctor puts it this way: "When the wheels fall off, you round up the usual suspects."

The suspects include common ailments such as infections, heart problems, strokes, and digestive diseases, but they most definitely include drug side effects. Where we have trouble is when there have been a lot of recent drug changes (so we don't know which suspect to round up) or if, as with Mr. Scarlatti, we don't even know he's on the medication. This is what I mean by obscure.

The more medication an elderly person is taking, the more difficult the doctor's job becomes. Blood levels of some drugs can change as a result of starting another one. Drug effects can crop up because another medication changes kidney or liver function, and so previously stable medicine is suddenly circulating at higher blood levels. The only way to find out if an old person's "going off" is caused by a medication is to stop the medications, very carefully, one at a time. Where there are two drugs, this trial-and-error process of reducing the dose and stopping each one in sequence may take a few weeks. Where there are six, well…

When a useless but potentially harmful medicine is tossed into the already complicated life of a Dave Scarlatti, it adds one more reason for him not to be quite his usual self. I think I'm as good as most ordinary doctors at figuring out what that reason is when there is a crisis of function, and I find it very difficult indeed. Most of the time, obscure, function-impairing drug effects look like a worsening of dementia or the result of advancing age. We can miss them easily.

Again, there is an the important difference between prevention based on common sense and prevention based on an imaginary mechanism. Yes, we should teach children not to get into strangers' cars. We should find out how deep the water is before we dive in. And regular exercise makes a person stronger and more flexible, so it makes sense to exercise regularly, to a reasonable level. And not just because it feels good (I dispute this, by the way, but I realize I'm in a minority); we can expect to function a little bit better with better strength and flexibility, and that *could* lead to not falling the next time somebody bumps into us. This is prevention, as it should be practiced.

But the fragile elderly live in an evidence-free zone; noncommonsense prevention with drugs makes no sense whatsoever. They suffer consequences that are hard to recognize and can destroy independence and capability for the rest of their lives. And we have to ask, What are we trying to prevent?

I hope in this discussion of prevention that I have pointed out a few disturbing cracks in the foundation of belief in preventing illness in fragile old people through certain kinds of behavior that we have come to believe are healthy. Our belief in prevention in these folks causes all sorts of glaring problems. In the next chapter I want to look at three things I see regularly where fragile people end up with a lot more than just theoretical trouble.

# 4 Three Blind Dice
## Examples of Prevention as a Gamble

### GWYN MEREDITH

Mr. Meredith was seventy-seven and appeared perfectly healthy when I first met him many years ago. He was one of my office patients and was handed over to a colleague when I left office practice to care for the elderly at home. He seemed made of iron in those days, in spite of a life that would have killed a lot of people off many times over.

He only attended a few years of grade school and began working in his native Wales as a teenager. He loved to describe rock-throwing fights with other children, his twelve-hour days as a farm laborer, and his later life as a coal miner. In particular I remembered his description of lunch in the mine: melted bacon fat soaked up with bread. Big quantities. More recently, when he was a car salesman and then after he retired, I knew he regularly bellied up to a breakfast of sausages and eggs; lunch of several white-bread sandwiches full of meat, butter, and mayonnaise; and dinner of meat and potatoes. He covered everything with salt, and in the unlikely event that any vegetable except potato appeared on his plate, he would melt a couple of tablespoons of butter over the top of it.

A few years into my home care practice I got a call from Mr. Meredith's daughter. The old man, now in his mideighties, had slowed down. In fact, his memory wasn't what it used to be, and his daughter and her husband had had to move him into their basement because he wasn't looking after himself properly in his apartment. The son-in-law was a pharmacist, a fitness enthusiast, and a believer in healthy eating. You can imagine the kind of difference of opinion that arose between him and my former patient.

Recently, the daughter told me, her dad had begun losing weight. Short and broad across the shoulders, Mr. Meredith had always weighed 185 pounds. And he wasn't fat. But in the six months since moving in with her family, he was down to below 150, didn't look all that great, and was spending less and less time outside or upstairs with her and the kids.

I took him back on as a patient and did my usual evaluation. I couldn't find anything much different from what I had known about Mr. Meredith many years previously. He was still hard as a rock, and all his systems appeared to be functioning perfectly well, with the exception of his brain, which was showing some short-term memory loss.

A bit baffled about the unexplained weight loss, I was all set to send him to an internal medicine geriatrics specialist for a more thorough going-over when, running late one afternoon, I pulled up for my visit at his house around 6 PM. Gwyn Meredith wasn't in his basement apartment but was upstairs having dinner with the family. I apologized for interrupting them and asked if it would be okay to check his blood pressure quickly (it had been a little low on a couple of previous occasions, especially when he stood up, though he was on no medication at all).

The dinner I saw on the table surprised me a little: it consisted entirely of vegetables. I recognized sliced tofu on the side of each plate, a big pile of bean sprouts, and something that appeared to be fried hummus. No saltshaker in sight.

The next time I spoke to Mr. Meredith, he was alone downstairs. He described his son-in-law's dietary ideas and admitted that now that he was having trouble getting out, he really wasn't eating very much at all. I arranged to meet with his daughter and her husband, and through a combination of careful diplomacy and professionally based bullying, I convinced them that the old man needed a different kind of food from what he was getting at home.

The introduction of judicious amounts of Mr. Meredith's preferred foods (doughnuts, pepperoni sausage, salt in a shaker, and red meat with a generous rind of fat around it) coincided with a gradual improvement in weight and a significant change in his mood and function. His blood pressure also stopped dropping when he stood up.

THIS CHAPTER LOOKS at several situations that I see in my practice over and over again. There are lots of examples of how old people in the real world routinely get into specific trouble because of efforts to prevent illness, but I'm going to focus on three of the ones most familiar to me.

The first is low blood pressure. *High* blood pressure is one of the oldest and most completely documented risk factors in medicine. Everybody knows about it. When we imagine a doctor, we may visualize the blood pressure cuff, a stethoscope, and a reassuring expression on the professional face designed to counter our reflex anxiety at the unpleasant things that might happen before we get out the door.

But high blood pressure has an ugly flip side in many of my patients. *Low* blood pressure is dangerous, very common, hard to detect, and pretty well guaranteed whenever doctors follow any of several preventive clinical guidelines. And low blood pressure is one of the most common causes of falls and injuries in old people.

A few groups of drugs, all of them also used to treat high blood pressure (they are, that is, effective at lowering blood pressure) have become best-practice treatment in preventing more than one health problem. Heart failure, heart attack, and diabetes all list one or several of these drugs among the treatments *required* to prevent these conditions' recurrence or resulting complications. Like diabetes and heart failure, heart attack is now defined by a test. All anybody wheeled through the doors of an emergency room or treated in a doctor's office has to do to fall into one of these disease categories is to "test positive": echocardiogram for heart failure, troponin for heart attack, and hemoglobin A1C for diabetes. If all of these tests are positive, you "have" all three diseases and typically get the full nine yards, potentially four or five separate drugs that all lower blood pressure.

When doctors are making up their minds whether somebody is going to get any or all of these medicines, there are some potent reinforcements to following the rules. Specialists will prescribe according to guidelines unless there is an obvious reason not to. Family physicians receive patients with specialists' recommendations and assume these well-informed doctors know best. Changes to guideline-mandated prescriptions are made at the doctor's peril; the patient's safety (and the doctor's) are understood to rely on sticking to those rules.

The trick with low blood pressure is that elderly people tend to have it anyway, independent of medication. But there are several special dangers that can result in low blood pressure–driven disasters, even when everyone does the job properly and has the best of intentions. One is that low blood pressure in old people may be intermittent and may be hard to detect.

Everything slows down with aging, including the speed of nerve impulses. The nerve impulses that keep the blood pressure up are the ones involved in the autonomic nervous system, particularly the sympathetic ("fight or flight") side of that system. Most feeling and movement involves our conscious brain, but the autonomic nervous system looks after built-in automatic patterns of response inherited from ancestors that go way back to primitive animals. The fight or flight response, driven by adrenaline, exists in everything from birds to baboons and is very familiar to us as part of our daily experience. And it happens whether we want it to or not. Think about how you feel when something really frightens you: your heart beats faster, you breathe a little more quickly, and you feel a sense of jumpiness and extra alertness or vigilance.

One of the effects of this fight or flight pattern is to push blood up into the brain. This happens when we're scared, but the sympathetic autonomic nervous system also adjusts blood flow when there's a sudden change in position, by clamping down the arteries, making the heart beat faster, and bumping up the blood pressure to get blood, with its oxygen, where it needs to go in a heartbeat or two. But the autonomic nervous system ages along with everything else.

Most people have experienced a "head rush" from standing up suddenly after being in a crouch for a minute or two. This is a minor version of what happens when an old person stands up suddenly. Nothing is perfect, and even in young, healthy people the autonomic nervous system takes a few moments to move enough blood around to get the brain what it needs. But in old people it takes longer, sometimes a lot longer. One of life's benign ironies is that the average old person takes a long time to get into an upright position but still sometimes stands up faster than the old system can respond to. It is a well-known result of normal aging that blood pressure drops with standing up and sometimes stays low for a few moments.

There are a couple of possible results. One is the geriatric version of the head rush, usually experienced as dizziness. If the blood pressure drop is a little more dramatic or it lasts a little longer, an old person can actually faint. Often when this happens, the story we hear is that there was a fall, and the elderly person may not even be aware of having had the experience. "I must have tripped," is the typical report.

This drop in blood pressure with a change in position only happens with the change in position, of course. In other words it's intermittent. For that reason it may be hard to detect. In the two most common situations where we take blood pressure, the drop can easily be missed. Situation number one is in the doctor's office, sitting on the examining table, where even a very frail, very old, thin person has had time for her blood pressure to adjust to normal if it ever does. Situation number two, maybe a little more dangerous, occurs in the hospital, where many routine blood pressures are taken lying down. A blood pressure drop with position change is going to be missed in this situation, too.

Heart attacks happen when the important arteries that carry blood directly to the heart muscle get blocked. But if those arteries are just partly obstructed, angina can occur. Textbook angina is chest pain that happens when you exert yourself. But it isn't always textbook. We saw an example of a diagnosis of angina in a not-so-typical situation when the heart specialist treated David Scarlatti for angina even though the pain everyone thought he had occurred at rest (and even though in fact he didn't have any pain at all). And one problem with the diagnosis of angina in old people is that often there is sluggish blood flow to the heart muscle, especially with exercise, without any pain. Sometimes the only result of that slow blood flow is a drop in blood pressure. The heart pump, which is just barely doing its job when a slow-moving elderly person is resting or walking around at his usual pace, gets faced with the demand of, for example, going up of flight of stairs and just can't deliver the goods because the arteries don't provide enough oxygen.

Here again we've got an old person whose blood pressure might be completely normal, even standing up. But if that person has to hurry up stairs for some reason, a drop in blood pressure might give her dizziness or even make her pass out. A frail arthritic person in a hurry can't afford dizziness, let alone a faint. Next frame: we're picking up the pieces at the bottom of the stairway.

Another thing that ages, like the autonomic nervous system, is sensation. Old people smell less and taste less than when they were younger, and they also don't experience thirst in the same way the rest of us do. In Chapter 3 Dick Halstadt refused to leave his sweatbox apartment, refused to stop his dehydrating water pill, and refused to drink liquids. One of the most common causes of low blood pressure is low blood volume, commonly known as dehydration. Nursing homes today make a project of giving residents lots of fluid in the summer, which is for sure a good idea because very old people get dehydrated as a result of not getting thirsty. This was one of the reasons Dick Halstadt had his fall. Even a thirsty frail person might not get enough fluid because they can't get out, there is not enough help at home, or they just forget.

And then something as apparently okay as eating a big healthy meal can drop the floor out from under somebody's blood pressure. Digestion is pretty dynamic, and when a load of corned beef and cabbage with hot mustard arrives at the stomach, blood circulation takes immediate notice. Blood flow is switched from everywhere else to the stomach and the bowel to carry the nutrients off to where they're needed. But there's only so much blood to go around. A blood pressure crash after somebody eats dinner may not matter much until that somebody gets up quickly, especially if dinner included a couple of glasses of wine.

The problem with intermittent low blood pressure in old people is that when doctors measure blood pressure, everything looks just fine. The HYVET study mentioned in Chapter 3 is being widely publicized, and the result will inevitably be more blood pressure–lowering prescriptions for more old people. But that apparently reasonable, guidelines-driven preventive medical care in which an old person might get multiple blood pressure–lowering drugs will nearly always, in my experience, put that blood pressure down to borderline low. Even an elderly-savvy prescribing doctor, trying to balance the benefit of prevention against the risk of side effects, may test the blood pressure sitting and standing and be reassured that there are no important side effects. But in the end she's just setting the frail old person up for the next unexpected intermittent drop in blood pressure.

In other words, when conscientious prescribers go looking for low blood pressure as the result of too much medication, it may not be there, because it only exists when the patient stands up quickly, on a hot day, when the heart isn't pumping properly, after a big meal, or with several of the above. That is, it exists in all sorts of perfectly common situations that are definitely going to happen sooner or later but that still will be missed.

Drug-industry TV ads love to scare us into going to the doctor by talking about high blood pressure as the silent killer. *Low* blood pressure would get my vote for that title in my population of old people. We can talk sagely about balancing the risks of preventing high blood pressure against the benefits, but once we really understand that there are no benefits, it's a little hard to justify any risk. And low blood pressure in a frail old person is a big risk.

The drug industry and academics carefully add up how many fewer hip fractures old people have when they take their drugs for osteoporosis, or bone thinning. But you break bones when you fall, and falling happens when old people get dizzy or faint, which happens when their blood pressure drops. Given the choice, I very carefully stop blood pressure–lowering preventive drugs and then take my chances with old bones as they are.

MY NEXT EXAMPLE of harm to the elderly from medical preventive practices usually occurs in the hospital, but not always. Over the past decade or so, understandable, well-intentioned zeal for prevention has resulted in special vigilance about swallowing, of all things. The professionals trained in this area—occupational therapists and speech language pathologists, primarily—work in hospitals and in the community and sometimes see people at home. The problem they are trying to prevent occurs when people who have trouble swallowing breathe in fluid, resulting in a kind of pneumonia. This can be serious, but what we do to prevent it can be a problem, too. A quick example may help here.

Daisy Neall was a tiny woman, ninety-two years old, living in subsidized senior citizens' housing operated by the Presbyterians. She fell walking down the hall to the laundry, though why she was doing this wasn't clear, since she had not been doing her own laundry for at least two years because of a worsening memory. Her right foot was crazily twisted around to the right when the ambulance arrived, indicating a broken hip, and she was taken to the hospital to have it repaired.

I first heard about the hospital admission and took over her care on the hospital ward three days after the surgery. She seemed to be doing just fine. Daisy had always been healthy; never married, she had spent a breathtakingly uneventful fifty years as an insurance secretary. Gradually losing her memory didn't seem to change her sensible, reverent approach to life much. As she lost independence, assistance had been provided at home.

Alert for the almost inevitable complications of being in the hospital, I wasn't surprised when Daisy became delirious about ten days after her surgery. Delirium is toxic confusion caused by pretty well any illness having a bad effect on an already demented brain. Rounding up the usual suspects, I realized she had become dehydrated. A blood test also confirmed there was not enough water in her system (the sodium was high). When I wrote in the orders, "Push oral fluids," I got a call an hour later from the nurse to say that they couldn't do this.

Apparently, three or four days before, a nursing student had heard Daisy sputter while swallowing her skim milk in an awkward position in bed. Within forty-five minutes an occupational therapy swallowing assessment had been performed, which Daisy failed with flying colors. "Thickened liquids" was the professional's response. Over the past few days my patient had been given an artificially thickened goo in place of milk, juice, and water. When I asked her about it, she said she hated the stuff and so had quit drinking.

We had quite a battle. Just as the occupational therapist was about to insist on referrals to several medical specialists, Daisy, who was having a relatively good day, sitting on the edge of her bed, grabbed a glass of orange juice off her roommate's tray and downed it convincingly in front of all of us. I was able to talk the team into a careful trial of regular fluid. Daisy did just fine. The delirium slowly cleared, and she made it home.

It is very difficult to bend the rules in hospitals, for some pretty good reasons. Swallowing assessments and the resulting treatment with thickened liquids are an example of why I advocate weighing priorities before deciding to clamp a guidelines-driven, textbook preventive "cure" onto someone who might not tolerate it. I don't always win the battles.

MY LAST EXAMPLE of how elderly people get into trouble because of preventive rules is much more general. I wonder how many readers of this book have eaten a nursing home meal. Since I confined my practice to seeing individual old people in their homes, I haven't seen as many patients harmed by ridiculous dietary rules, but it still happens. In my opinion the general perception that "eating healthy" never hurt anybody is dangerous nonsense where fragile older people are concerned.

Gwyn Meredith's story may strike some people as funny, but he couldn't have lost much more weight without getting into more serious trouble as a result of malnutrition. He could have died—and I believe others have—of what is now referred to as "orthorexia," also known as excessively healthy eating. Hardly healthy.

A blunted sense of smell and taste is a normal characteristic of aging and occurs very slowly. Many older people compensate by eating more strongly flavored food. This tendency results in a clash between "healthy eating" as most of us understand it and healthy eating from the point of view of an old person with a lot of health problems. Healthy eating for older people is eating what they *enjoy,* period. Here's why.

We are told we are what we eat, and we believe this. Healthy eating is as unquestioned as the evils of cigarette smoking and the benefits of brushing your teeth. Information about it is also well disseminated; everybody knows raw vegetables are good and fat is bad. And healthy eating, of course, is *scientific.*

We have seen that there are problems with science based on randomized controlled trials, especially where old people are concerned. But the science backing up the benefits of a healthy diet is much worse. It is, for openers, impossible to do a placebo-controlled trial of eating. You have to look at the results of questionnaires asking people what they've had for dinner over the last few years and then look at whether there is a difference in how long the ones who have been enjoying turnips and oat bran live compared with people who eat mostly burgers and fries.

There is a subculture of people in the health professions who are skeptical analysts of scientific evidence. They believe that science must be of the very best quality before we accept it as a basis for action. Many members of this crowd are internal medicine specialists in clinical pharmacology and statisticians, and I tend to agree with them.

When confronted with badly done, biased, irrelevant research about drugs, these people routinely and properly howl with protest. But I never hear a peep out of any of them on the subject of the dreadful quality of evidence supporting healthy eating. So pervasively are we socialized on this subject that even the most nihilistic science skeptics still happily live their dietary lives according to one or another of the national Guidelines for Healthy Eating. Drug industry: evil! Healthy eating: good! There is something other than science operating here.

Even if the science supporting healthy eating were good, there wouldn't be any basis for believing in prevention in the population of fragile old people. But the science is bad, so there must be some other reason why we do the kind of thing the son-in-law did to Mr. Meredith. Here's what I think: the basis for restricted-salt, low-fat, no-trans-fat, natural-food, high-fiber, no-sugar, organically grown eating among elderly people is simply cultural. If we want to have fish on Friday, great, as long as we don't do it to improve our health.

Although there are obese elderly, it's very much more common to see older patients who are losing weight. The more dependent, medicated, forgetful, and immobile someone becomes, the likelier they are not to eat enough. Being cultural creatures, we respond to their malnutrition culturally, in the guise of science. No salt, only fat-free ice cream, and desserts with all the sugar sucked out of them. This to prevent high blood pressure, heart attacks, and diabetes. Living at home, an old person may still have some faint hope of getting food with some flavor. But not always. Take a seat in the dining room of your local nursing home, however, and ask yourself if what they put in front of the people who live there makes you want to come back tonight for dinner.

I don't mean to malign nutritionists or nursing home chefs. Physicians are as guilty as anybody of handing out misinformation about eating. But this is beside the point. If we were talking about whether to watch golf or hockey on TV (something that had no serious impact on anybody's life), it wouldn't make any difference if we held an irrational belief that seeing too many golf games results in cancer of the pancreas. But old people need tasty food to maintain their body weight and general well-being. If they don't get it because we insist on giving them food that tastes to them like boiled cardboard, and they become malnourished, we are the ones to blame.

This problem of encouraging malnutrition with "healthy eating" leaves aside altogether the quality-of-life question. If I ever make it into my eighties, you can be damn sure that I won't be giving up life's most consistent satisfaction for any reason. Your usual fragile elderly person's daily life doesn't necessarily snap and crackle with uninterrupted sensual excitement. Making sure they get great-tasting food isn't just about preventing malnutrition.

Preventing heart attacks, preventing choking, and being careful about what you eat all have their place. It's when we do these things according to rules and procedures, with no particular regard for people for whom those rules and procedures don't work—and to whom they sometimes cause harm—that we start having real trouble.

The next chapter discusses the consequences of modern health care's other priority, rescue, on the elderly. Prevention leads to medication, and rescue leads straight to one of the worst places a fragile elderly person can be: the hospital.

# 5  The Cathedrals of Crisis
Rescue and the Hospital

**MITCHELL ACKERMAN**

Not all my fragile, homebound patients are old. One of the younger ones, Mitch, was a thin, bearded, long-haired man of about forty with terribly crippling multiple sclerosis. He was also resilient and had a sense of humor. It was obvious that he smoked marijuana regularly, and I would see some shady characters coming and going from his place when I visited. But I never felt anything from Mitch but direct honesty and a breathtaking absence of self-pity. He was a lovely man.

Mitch needed help every day getting from his bed to his wheelchair. He had also developed openings in his skin where his bones stuck out. Months of home care nurses' superhuman efforts couldn't heal these pressure sores in his apartment. An expensive pressure-relieving bed would have done the trick, but there wasn't enough money for one, and so finally there was no choice but to admit him to hospital to try to heal the sores. I did the medical care while nurse experts worked on the wounds.

One morning when I visited, I saw a referral to a psychiatrist on the chart. The hospital social worker explained that Mitch had given some strange answers to straightforward questions about diet, and the team of a nutritionist, nurses, and rehabilitation people on the ward were concerned that he might not be competent to make decisions. Although I am quite experienced at evaluating decision-making ability, and although I knew perfectly well that Mitch's strange answers were just his unusual sense of humor, hospital policy required a psychiatric evaluation if there was any question about decision-making capability. Team members understood what I said to them, but policy is policy. We don't make the rules.

Mitch gave the psychiatrist the same ironic song and dance he'd given the nutritionist, with the result that he was given an antipsychotic tranquilizer and was declared incapable. The psychiatrist noticed abnormalities on a chest x-ray (of which I was well aware, and which were trivial) and recommended consulting a respiratory specialist. The treatment of his pressure sores was complicated because his movements were frozen by the antipsychotic drug.

The respiratory specialist ordered breathing tests that took two weeks to complete, and other consultations were triggered by those results. When the pressure sores finally began to heal, Mitch couldn't leave the hospital because there were more consultations and tests to be done, and he had been deemed incapable of discharging himself against advice. I struggled to contact everyone involved, tried to arrange meetings, and did everything else I could to get him out of there, but before I could, he contracted hospital-bug pneumonia, which the infectious disease specialists couldn't treat. Eventually, after multiple team meetings involving a hospital ethicist, it was decided not to admit Mitch to the intensive care unit on a respirator, and Mitch died.

The cost of his hospital admission was thirty times the cost of the bed that would have healed the sores at home.

## MARTHA CLEAVER

When I was still looking after people in hospital, seventy-eight-year-old Mrs. Cleaver, a kidney-failure patient, got very short of breath at home on the weekend. When I went to see her, I could see she was in heart failure. I gave some injected treatment, which didn't help. Although Mrs. Cleaver spent many hours at the hospital every week on a kidney machine, she had always felt strongly that she didn't want to be admitted (spend the night there, that is), having had a terrible experience in hospital once before. "Better-off dead," she said.

So we faced a difficult choice: at this point, it looked as though the only way to get her comfortable was to find out what was wrong quickly and treat it if we could. We finally agreed that it would be worse for her to continue to feel the way she did than to face her fear of being mistreated in the hospital. After an evaluation in the emergency room she was admitted with a diagnosis of pulmonary embolism (lung clot) and treated in an intensive-care unit. Her three-times-weekly kidney-machine treatment continued.

I saw her every day. She hated being in the hospital but was improving. Still under the care of the hospital specialists, she was moved outside intensive care. Unfortunately the improvement was short-lived. At my visit one Sunday morning, the shortness of breath had come back, and the attending specialists were in the process of trying to figure out whether she would benefit from being back in the intensive care unit. As I explained what was going on, Mrs. Cleaver said, "Oh my God, doctor, I think the breathing is really getting worse now!" I could see it was. The physical findings in my examination were dramatic and bad. Now she was really working to take every breath and was horribly afraid. I called for help, and in a minute a senior medical resident and the intensive care doctor on call came out of the elevator.

It's hard for me to describe my profound mixed feelings. Those doctors and everyone else did their work very well. A portable x-ray machine appeared and films were taken; the doctors made their quick decisions and gave orders; medication was injected. Mrs. Cleaver had a breathing tube in her throat twenty-five seconds after it was needed. All my years of training told me how well the difficult technical job was being done. I was filled with pride: these people are really good!

But at the same time I could see we were fighting a losing battle, and my patient's last experience on earth was probably going to be panic, with a plastic tube in her throat and a lot of people rushing around manipulating equipment as if she herself weren't there. Her eyes were wide open and jumping from side to side. With everything we tried to do, the specialists looked to me to help decide whether to proceed. At each step, remembering Mrs. Cleaver's desire to get better again and knowing the lung clot had been improving, I couldn't bring myself to order a stop. I held her hand and explained as best I could.

She died after about ninety minutes of our best efforts.

PEOPLE WHO LIKE to be optimistic about the state of the medical system are pleased at statistics showing that prevention is working. And, they tell us, when and if it doesn't work, we are ready with a sophisticated, state-of-the-art system to rescue people when they do get into trouble in spite of living right. The more complicated, the worse, the more dangerous, and the more horrifying the problem, the more sophisticated and rigorous our solutions. And the most sophisticated and rigorous solutions live in hospitals. The system is designed to match the awfulness of the problem to the exceptional effectiveness of the hospital solution. Well, rescue of that kind isn't what fragile elderly patients need.

Old people regularly come out of the hospital in trouble. Why is that? Don't the doctors—we're talking about the big university specialists here—know what they're doing? Did a pharmacist make a mistake? Are the residents and medical students incompetent or unsupervised? Or are some patients just too sick to be helped?

Most of the time it's none of the above. What I see coming off the assembly line of state-of-the-art hospital care is a frail old person with complicated needs who, instead of rolling out onto the loading dock as a perfect product, got mangled somewhere in the machinery. And part of the problem is that that efficient hospital production line *works*. It's as effective as a stainless-steel trap. Doctors, policies and procedures, and most of the other people and processes that make the wheels go around inside a hospital are very good indeed at following rules and minimizing risk.

Rescue as a concept is driven by the powerful and admirable human tendency to do good things for others: if someone is in trouble, we rush in and help. This presumes that the help we offer is wanted and will be effective, and it usually is both of these things. The rescue idea captures our imagination in crisis: a car accident, somebody who can't breathe, a very sick child, injury on the job. We sit on the edge of our chairs with excitement.

Anyone who has ever really needed to be rescued requires no convincing. We want to be damn sure that when we push the 911 panic button, help is on its way fast.

Most people are familiar with the critical care side of the medical system: the sort of stuff that happens in those sophisticated high-tech hospitals. We fortunate ones who have never had to use it ourselves understand what it feels like through doctor, hospital, firefighter, and emergency-room TV shows. And the best ones only help me make my point. One of the reasons I liked ER, for example, was that there was nearly always a confused elderly person drifting around, if for no other reason than to relieve the tense and thrilling excitement of bleeding crash victims and the love lives of the fascinating doctors and nurses.

What about those fragile old people wandering, apparently lost, in the hospital? The kind of crisis they have just isn't the kind that the critical care system is designed to rescue people from. That crisis tends to come at us looking like a collapse in function. Mum can't get from her bed to the bathroom anymore. Dad is getting really confused, and we can't leave him alone, even for an hour. If this kind of change in function happens quickly, if we panic, or if we honestly just have no idea what to do, our response may be hospital, via what I call the 911 panic button. The rescue system is waiting with open arms. It will arrive with a lot of noise and whip the elderly person out the door, into an ambulance, to the emergency room, and into the hospital. There, the incompatibilities between that old person's real needs and the resources of the critical care system are plain for everyone to see.

Rescue as it is practiced today is necessary, wonderful when it's really needed, and usually quite beautifully done. But trying to rescue an old person in crisis using the usual tools of the critical care system is like trying to evacuate a crowded theater by shouting "Fire!" It is bound to make things worse, because it just plain doesn't get the nature of the problem.

Critical care rescue's limitations for a troubled old person are as real as the ones we saw with prevention. And they come from the same place: guidelines-driven, scientific evidence–based health care. A paramedic may recognize some similarity to his grandfather when he arrives to treat an elderly man who has made the mistake of telling his neighbor he is feeling dizzy and weak. The guidelines driving the paramedic tell him to stabilize the old guy and get him into the hospital. But what the old man really needs is a couple of extra hours of home support next week while a capable home care health professional finds out what's wrong with him.

Modern rescue guidelines are rigid and well researched. We wouldn't have them any other way. Nobody wants the paramedic who is supposed to recognize a dangerous health crisis and get the person in for treatment wasting time being a social worker. No issue: a social worker he typically isn't. But once that paramedic has been and gone, taking the fragile old person with him, it isn't possible anymore to do what the patient really needed, which would have involved a home care family doctor, a nurse, and probably a social worker to get him home support, analyze his crisis, and try to make the crisis go away.

Another big limitation of critical care rescue is also one of its greatest strengths: it is available twenty-four hours a day, seven days a week. It is the venue of default in a medical system that hasn't figured out that to properly help fragile older people, we need to meet their needs 24/7. In some communities, especially late at night and on the weekend, it may be the only light on in town. So when *anything* is wrong, there just isn't any choice but to call for the kind of help we don't really need.

That emergency response, which, according to procedural rules, may include firefighters and police officers, is set up to deal effectively with serious health problems that need fast diagnosis and quick treatment. This means that whenever the first-response paramedic identifies a significant illness on the scene, the person who apparently has it will be transported to the emergency room.

Designed and equipped for rapid diagnosis and treatment, the emergency room and its people function like a complicated piece of machinery. The ER is like a hospital on steroids. Several diagnoses may be made inside the first thirty minutes, each leading to actions that are required based on hospital policy. These might be emergency treatments like an intravenous line or oxygen, dozens of blood tests (the results of which may trigger other guidelines), tests and imaging to evaluate heart function or scan the brain or lungs (also resulting in diagnoses and other pathways), referrals to all sorts of experts or teams (which could include psychiatry, sexual assault consultants, surgery, or the intensive care unit), placing of special monitoring equipment, including catheters in the heart, and many, many types of drug treatment together with the need to monitor their results.

When a patient in my practice is sent to the hospital by ambulance (usually because of a change in function and need for increased support that somebody believes they can't handle) I'm usually not called. I will first hear of the whole thing three or four days after the fact. A completely unexpected hospital specialist's report on a person I thought was at home slides out of the fax machine, say. The poor receiving people at the emergency room would have had to deal with a person who can't walk, who can't tell them why she is there, and who lights up like a Christmas tree when they start doing all the usual investigations. Urine is infected. Blood oxygen is low. Heart attack blood test is slightly elevated. Kidney function is abnormal. Heart pump function is not good. Blood sugar is elevated. Et cetera, et cetera. With no background or anything else to guide them, hospital admission to "sort things out" is inevitable.

On any given day most of my patients would have all those "abnormalities" found in the emergency room, and they are perfectly harmless findings. I call this the "Velcro phenomenon," which causes the average elderly person to stick when she hits the hospital. None of the problems identified there is typically unknown to the family doctor, home care nurse, or others working in the community, and most of them are stable. This means that while they are real problems, they aren't causing any trouble with function or comfort at the moment, and we're keeping an eye on them.

The problem with critical care rescue, the ER, and the hospital has nothing to do with the people who work there. And if things didn't run according to rules, emergency rooms would be even more horrifying nightmares than they already are. The reason they don't work for the fragile elderly is that they need something completely different than what the ER is so good at providing.

The professionals working in the ER typically have criteria for whom they can "treat and release" (send home). Fragile elderly people almost never meet those criteria and so are admitted to hospital. But the hospital and the elderly are one another's worst nightmares. This is because the hospital's purpose and elderly people's needs are on completely different planets.

Dr. Robert Mendelsohn, in his book *Confessions of a Medical Heretic*, starts his chapter on hospitals this way: "A hospital is like a war." Although Mendelsohn was writing in the 1970s, these wonderful centers of technologic excellence still have a dark side today, at times blacker than ever. Hospitals stock thousands of dangerous drugs, harbor bacteria found nowhere else on earth and for which there is no cure, and rely heavily on—celebrate, in fact—experts and machinery so specialized and complicated that virtually nobody really understands their function. Also encountered frequently enough to become something nobody finds out of the ordinary in every hospital is death.

A friend very familiar with the medical system said to me recently, "Sometimes the only way an old person can get out of the hospital is to die." How could the kind of place we trust to help us when we're in trouble, and where the most highly respected health professionals work, *trap* elderly people, as my friend was implying?

Part of the reason is that once in the hospital (because of the rules in place in the emergency room), old people lose flexibility, strength, and confidence over the many days the hospital may take to sort out their problems. Never mind that many of these problems are unsolvable—many are already known to non-hospital professionals, and many of them have already been investigated at least once.

The longer an older person is in the hospital, the more Kafkaesque the situation becomes and the lower the person's chances of getting out unharmed. Clinical guidelines that physicians more or less follow in their offices become "clinical pathways"—unvarying policies and procedures—in the hospital. These exist for nearly all the ordinary problems people in the hospital usually have, and they automatically snap like leghold traps in response to specific triggers. People who work in hospitals have no choice but to follow these pathways. Old people bristle with the triggers that set off these traps and simply can't be in the hospital without accumulating dozens of metaphorical jagged iron jaws all over and around them.

These clinical pathways, like the rules of diagnosis and treatment designed for prevention with medication, are of course scientific. Evidence based.

But for fragile old people the system goes back again and again, like a recursive computer program, trying to fix the eventually unfixable problems they have, because the hospital's scientific procedures are designed for cure. The rules are rarely broken, and for old people they form the walls of a maze that sometimes only leads toward its own center. Three days in bed, with the accompanying loss of strength, flexibility, and confidence, plus the whole cascade of consequences of unavoidable hospital guidelines, leads to weeks and weeks lying in a hospital bed, with less and less chance of ever returning home with each passing day. I call the fragile elderly and the acute-care hospital a marriage made in hell: I'm no good for you; you're no good for me. We will deal with "you're no good for me" a little later. The hospital doesn't escape unharmed, either.

Mitch Ackerman was an example of a fragile person trapped in the hospital. Although not old, he shared most of the fragile elderly's characteristics. Care at home would have been possible and certainly would have been preferable, if the resources had been available. They weren't. And it would be hard to find fault with the hospital-ward team members, whose job descriptions included following hospital policies and procedures. They didn't make the rules, and they could be disciplined for deviating from them. Everybody did exactly what he or she was supposed to do.

The hospital Mitch died in also has a large and active "risk management" office. This is the part of hospital administration that sees to minimizing risk, both to patients and to the hospital. Paying attention to what could go wrong to prevent trouble later is important. What if a doctor or nurse in a hospital presents a patient with an important health decision and follows the patient's wishes, and then that patient dies? Next the family appears, lawyered up, insisting that their poor old relative had no idea what he was talking about. It is less risky to have a psychiatrist determine the mental capability of the patient if any question arises. And that's exactly what happened to Mitch Ackerman.

Now every doctor practicing on the staff of a properly regulated acute-care hospital is required to meet clinical guidelines. These are similar to the ones we've talked about for diagnosis and treatment: rules for responding to findings like a raised temperature, an abnormal blood test, an x-ray showing something that could be cancer, and certain kinds of infections. The rules exist partly so that bad, "loose-cannon" doctors of the old-fashioned style who used to swashbuckle around hospitals barking orders without explanation can't make crazy, irresponsible decisions that result in disasters.

Mitch's psychiatrist did the reasonable thing in a hospital context. He was worried that his patient might have some physical condition (apart from his multiple sclerosis) that was causing him to behave in a strange way. He reviewed the chart, and there was something wrong on the chest x-ray. He is a psychiatrist in the middle of a hospital filled with every imaginable kind of specialist. So he called the chest specialist. That specialist in today's regulated environment is not in a position to second-guess another expert, either. Even if she could somehow see a bigger picture than the x-ray of the patient's lungs (let's imagine she was for some reason on the same wavelength as Mitch's nutty ironic way of looking at the world), it simply would not have been her place to question a colleague in his area of expertise.

I've had many years of experience working with all sorts of doctors. Some of the most sensible, kind, and intuitive people I've ever met are highly focused medical specialists. Constrained by institutional rules, they must balance their instincts against their training and against those rules. I know they lie awake at night second-guessing their decisions, as I do. Was I careful enough? Should I have done another test? Should I have spent a bit more time explaining things? Again, it's not the people who are the problem in hospitals.

And I am not advocating a return to the old-fashioned swash-buckling doctor and a culture of irresponsibility based on arro-gance. But regulation and consistency come at a price. My patient Mitch Ackerman paid it because it just wasn't possible to get him free from the hospital's machinery.

Rescue in crisis for old people means keeping their depen-dence from getting worse, keeping them comfortable, and keep-ing their daily function where it is. The hospital is the last place to diagnose, support, and deal with this kind of crisis.

But the picture as it suddenly presents itself to us is rarely that simple. I was filled with professional pride at the hospital's response to Martha Cleaver's crisis even as I cursed what was happening to her. With Martha even someone as wary as I am about a futile technical rescue found it irresistible, and she was therefore admitted to hospital. It was the lesser of two worri-some evils. But descent into more and more highly technical ef-forts to rescue someone is a certain kind of slippery slope. Only in retrospect do we realize that technical rescue was futile and perhaps even worse than nothing; we sometimes just can't see the wrongness of it coming until it's too late.

For an old person at home who is not coping well or is suddenly in trouble, the conventional rescue route involving the ambulance, the hospital, and specialists can appear, and be, quite compelling. The decision about what to do can be really difficult. And sometimes it has to be made quickly.

There are really two kinds of crises. One is an unexplained change in function caused by a minor health problem, as when Mrs. Bellamy from Chapter 1 woke up with the flu and couldn't get out of bed. The second is a serious, dangerous-looking illness that could be fatal. This second type of crisis also shows up as a change in function. A sudden, dangerous illness is no more likely to show its face as plainly as if it came off the pages of a textbook than any other health condition in an old person. But if we recognize it for what it is or looks as though it might be, the critical care rescue solution may appear extremely compelling. But it's still nearly always the wrong thing to do.

The huge majority of crises I see in practice are of the first kind: a significant change in function probably based on a minor illness. The first thing to do in the face of such a change is to round up the usual suspects: common minor crises. These include a common simple infection (bladder or chest infection, usually); a little, unrecognized injury; dehydration; or some kind of change in medication. The other important thing is to support function until the dust clears—until you know whether you're dealing with a permanent change or not.

Supporting function isn't rocket science. Mrs. Bellamy from Chapter 1 got more home support for a while because while she had the flu, she couldn't get out of bed and was a little more

confused than usual. Someone else who normally looks after their own housecleaning and cooking might need help with
those things, usually temporarily.

Most of the time the crisis simply goes away on its own.
Other times a simple medical workup turns up one of the usual
suspects, which is treated. Primary care evaluation and treatment at home is the proper handling of that first, common kind
of crisis.

*Wrong* handling of a common crisis is either to assume it is
just part of getting old and start planning for transfer to a nursing home or to become overwhelmed by the sudden change in
care needs (the need to nurse somebody in bed for a few days and
to provide meals for a week or so, all without much warning).
The first mistake directs the old person toward a nursing home,
and the second one pushes the critical care panic button and
leads to the Big Mistake of an unnecessary trip to the hospital.

The second kind of crisis, the sudden, dangerous illness kind,
is complicated by an important moral issue. Here's an example
to introduce this second, more urgent kind of crisis.

Difficult ninety-one-year-old Mrs. Chau was living in a fancy,
expensive assisted-living facility. She had kidney failure that was
not bad enough to need a kidney machine, very high blood pressure, smoker's lungs, and some dementia. The dementia had ex-
aggerated certain aspects of her personality, and she behaved as
if everything was pointless and depressing and then manipu-
lated everybody around her into trying to do something about it,
blaming them when, of course, they couldn't. That included me,
who had her on antidepressants.

Her family was at their wits' end trying to please the old lady
and at the same time trying to set limits on her demands, which
amounted to a desire to be forty years old again (I had trouble

finding fault with that). When I tried, as I usually do, to get her to tell me whom she would like to make health care decisions for her if she were ever unable to make them for herself, she listed her children and then told me one after another why each of them couldn't be trusted. Finally she said her sister was the one who should decide. When I called the sister, I discovered that she was also a very elderly lady who obviously had more than her own share of problems and who didn't feel up to being a substitute decision maker for her sister or anybody else. Both Mrs. Chau and her daughter, however, were very clear that she preferred not to go to the hospital if she could be treated at home.

In that advance directive semi-limbo, a nurse at the facility called one afternoon to tell me that Mrs. Chau was more confused than usual. My examination showed definite new congestive heart failure, which I treated with medication. A few days later my patient was worse. The heart failure was a bit better, but her blood pressure was falling, and she was more and more confused. The daughter confirmed that the family didn't want her to go to hospital unless it was "absolutely necessary." I started antibiotics in case chest infection was part of the problem. The next day Mrs. Chau was found on the floor, and when I rushed over to see her, she was semiconscious and quite short of breath and had low blood pressure. Although she wasn't saying anything coherent, she was terribly distressed, resisting my examination and moaning loudly. The daughter was there, very anxious and upset, and the elderly sister also arrived.

I could see in this situation an example of the second, more dramatic kind of crisis in an old person. But should she go to hospital? Damned if you do, damned if you don't. This chronically ill old lady with poorly functioning kidneys and lungs at the best of times was really in trouble. Trouble because she appeared to be dying, and trouble because she was obviously in awful emotional and physical distress. I sat the daughter and sister down and told them what I thought: it was *possible* that everything we were seeing was due to an infection, which in theory could be treated more aggressively and possibly be cured. Much likelier, I told them, Mrs. Chau had had a heart attack and, with both breathing trouble and low blood pressure, her chances of recovery were very poor. We could put her back into bed and make her comfortable with morphine, and I would expect her to die within a day or two. Or we could call an ambulance and see whether they could get her better at the hospital.

The daughter couldn't face the uncertainty of her mum staying in her home. She was, I understood, also subject to the second-guessing of her two high-powered brothers, both available only by phone, both very inclined to make sure we did everything we could. I called the emergency room, explained the whole situation to the doctor, and gave the paramedics my version of the story before they headed for the hospital, red lights and siren clearing the road in front of them.

Mrs. Chau died around midnight that night. Tests in emergency showed both heart attack and pneumonia.

When I am called urgently because someone like Mrs. Chau appears, more or less suddenly, to be in a lot of trouble, I can usually make some educated guesses about what is wrong and provide some idea of what is likely to happen. But it would be unusual for me to be really certain about the diagnosis. If in that circumstance we decide not to call for critical care rescue, then we face the prospect that someone we are responsible for and love will get worse and then possibly die at home, without our really knowing what happened. And we can see on the horizon—at the same time as we are trying to decide whether to pull out all the stops, call the ambulance, and try to find out what's wrong and fix it—how we will feel about not knowing what happened. Bad. Guilty. What if it was something we *could* have fixed? And how awful to face that question over and over for years and have buried the answer forever. But let's be perfectly clear about one thing: this is a problem for *us*, the survivors.

On the other side we have Mrs. Cleaver. She died terrified, knowing what was happening, in the middle of a panic-stations scene, unable to affirm anything, unable to ask anything, an object of technical attention with (except for helpless little me) everybody around her completely focused on their job. If circumstances had allowed, she could have died at home with her family around her, comforted by just the right amount of morphine and lots of love and reassurance. She could have said the things that needed saying. But that awful final experience was a problem for *her*. Her family, the nurses, and the doctors, including me, got to go home thinking, "We did our best."

The question to ask is whose interest is favored in these situations. The exact circumstances are always unique. But we who are making the decisions must be careful we don't misuse our power to decide. Whom are we looking after when we sacrifice comfort and kindness for technical heroics?

Often (and I did this with Mrs. Chau and her family) I just ask myself, "What would I do if this were my mum?" (My mum died many years ago.) Sometimes I just don't know the answer. But for the huge majority of potentially life-threatening crises in many elderly people, the people in my practice, transport to hospital for almost anything is both horrifying and futile. My decision for my own mum, if she couldn't make the decision herself, would be to keep her comfortable. But my mum isn't every mum—I happen to know that mine would have agreed completely with being kept comfortable. It could be different for someone with different values. It's very different if you can't get an urgent medical assessment at home. It's also different if for any reason you can't make somebody comfortable at home. Let's not forget, though, that in these critical situations the choice is made by people other than the old person herself: family, friends, nurses, and me. And I'm afraid the temptation is often overwhelming to spare *ourselves* the lingering question of whether something could have been done.

Both kinds of functional crisis in old people demand a careful evaluation of the possible causes. While there are exceptions, the default attitude for me is that my patients are better off at home. The decision of whether critical care rescue is a good idea or not is made by the patient or the people responsible for making decisions for her—with my advice if they want it and always with my reassurance that staying home is not abandonment. I'm there to help, to comfort, and to make the illness better if I can. And the hospital, however convinced we may be that it is the right place for a sick person, is nearly always the wrong place for someone who is dependent, near the end of life, and inclined to prefer kindness to the cutting edge of technology.

So what are we supposed to do about the marriage made in hell? The answer has nothing to do with fixing the way the hospital and the rest of the critical care rescue system does business. Everything I've ever observed suggests that that business gets done quite well most of the time. Regulation and consistency are absolutely necessary for many of the things that must be done in a hospital. The operating room must be as close to sterile as it is humanly possible to make it. A person who gets a temperature two days after an operation must be investigated and the cause identified.

But all that high-performance rigor and consistency doesn't work for the consistently oddball type of patient I'm responsible for in my practice. That person needs the thoughtful, creative, individual exercise of common sense and judgment that was the trademark of the very best of those unregulated, old-fashioned doctors. And many of my colleagues in hospitals have all that wisdom and more. It's just that when you work in a hospital, it's very hard indeed to use it sometimes. Very effective adherence to rules and wide discretion for exception just can't live in the same box.

My answer? Keep the Mitch Ackermans of the world away from the doors of the emergency room. Don't let the marriage made in hell happen in the first place. Care for them at home.

When my turn comes, spare me, please. Perform a technically exemplary cardiac-arrest resuscitation on an accident victim and instead quietly give me comfort medicine, hand-holding as long as I want it, honest tears, and snow-white lies. A gentle last experience on earth is just fine with me.

# 6 Falling Between the Cracks
## Geriatric NIMBYism

**KIRSTI SEPPANEN**

This lady was a patient from the beginning of my family practice in 1978. At that time, she lived with her retired carpenter husband in a tiny, perfect house in a low-rent downtown neighborhood and would get to my office via a two-hour bus ride. After her husband died, Mrs. Seppanen gradually developed arthritis and memory trouble, so she naturally fit into my home-visit practice when I left the office in 1993.

What a powerful character! She was tall and heavy and strong as a moose. Her huge gap-toothed smile or, when that failed, a tantrum in Finnish usually got her what she wanted. She was incredibly self-reliant. As immigrants in the 1940s, she and her husband bought their property for a few hundred dollars and built their house by hand. She did all her own cooking and canning, and although, as mobility and memory failed, she accepted help from friends and her church, she was very reluctant to admit home support workers, home care nurses, or any other helpers to her home. And she was absolutely adamant from day one that she would never go to a nursing home.

Her problems got worse. I would knock on the door and wait three or four minutes before eventually hearing the scrape of her walker and stumping of her shoes as she came to the door. Another thirty seconds to undo the five front door locks, and then she would give me a long, quizzical look over the safety chain as she tried to figure out who I was. It got harder and harder to convince her that she knew me and that I was the doctor.

A nephew from out of town arranged all sorts of consultations. An Alzheimer's clinic confirmed the diagnosis but couldn't change the memory loss. A rheumatologist confirmed the osteoarthritis but properly decided reconstructive surgery didn't make sense as long as she could walk. A mental health team was involved, and so was a long-term-care case manager and home care nurses to help with her leg ulcers. Eventually she allowed home support workers in to make meals and do the cleaning.

She had five or six crises. Once, she fell and was on the floor for twenty-four hours on the weekend. Another time she was terribly confused and wouldn't let anyone in. We had to break the lock on a window for me to see her, diagnose her urinary tract infection, and get her on medication. Each time, the community professionals insisted that she needed to go to the hospital or be admitted to a nursing home. Each time I suggested these things to her, she would pound her cane on the floor and shout, "No! I die *here!*"

There is no question in my mind that if I hadn't been seeing her at home and been available on call for crises at all hours, she would have been towed away to the hospital and would have died five times over, angry and bewildered in a nursing home. Instead, the home support worker found her dead in her bed one morning with a peaceful look on her face.

### HENRI BOISVERT OR TOO MANY COOKS FOR THE COOK

This man, a retired French-Canadian pea-soup-and-poutine chef, was a patient in a veterans' extended-care unit. He had pretty bad dementia from head injuries, a life of alcohol abuse, and strokes and was famous all over the hospital as a "screamer." He would shout for hours in a piercing tenor voice. Closing the windows and doors didn't make much difference. Nurses put deaf people in the room with him, and he drove even them crazy.

Before I started on the unit, a lot of different doctors, including a psychiatrist, had been prescribing for Henri. When I saw him for the first time, I heard that the shouting had stopped just a few weeks ago. Everybody was relieved. When I went to his room, he was being fed even though he was apparently fast asleep, and it seemed an awfully long time between breaths. Like about one every fifteen seconds.

Henri was taking four different drugs to settle his behavior. He had quieted down a little after each one was started but then slowly went back to his nonstop yelling. It seemed they had had trouble finding a family doctor for him, so the on-call physician or psychiatrist would always get called when his screaming became unbearable. Each doctor tried another drug, with the same result: things settled down but then got worse again. But nobody had stopped the drugs that didn't work. He was quiet all right, but by now most of his remaining brain cells were saturated with medication, and he was barely breathing.

After we slowly got rid of all four sedatives, Henri of course went back to shouting. It took a few months of trial and error to figure out that he was in pain but couldn't tell anybody; he had an overflowing, blocked bladder but couldn't tell anybody; and he was terrified of women, who made up nine out of ten of his care providers. These days he still shouts the odd time, and he is on one drug to control behavior, but things are a bit quieter.

OLD PEOPLE SUFFER because we overmedicate them in a well-intentioned attempt to improve their future. They get lost in a maze of technology when we misunderstand their relatively simple needs for care at home and try to rescue them when something goes wrong. But there is another problem our system visits on these folks. They fall between the cracks.

I've always found the phrase "falling between the cracks" ironic. We have a picture in our mind of small objects falling through cracks in a floor, say. But if you can fall *between* the cracks it has to mean there's nothing but cracks. And there are times when the medical system looks that way from the point of view of a typical old person I see every day.

Old people fall between the cracks in the medical system because we don't know when to say "enough!" We are afraid to abandon prevention and rescue because we believe in them, as we believe in the whole intellectual structure that produced them, but we understand perfectly well that somewhere along the road from full independent function to full dependence on others, prevention and rescue don't make sense, don't work anymore, and need to be abandoned in favor of something different. But where on that road is that supposed to happen?

This question can't be answered in the abstract any more than we can deal with any problems with the frail elderly in the abstract. But we will try and try to find abstract answers to big, important questions. It's just how we do business for some reason.

If we know our usual health solutions don't apply to these people, and yet it's unconscionable simply to abandon them, what are we supposed to do? Just about everybody in all corners of the health care system, from the most overarching administrator down to an ordinary front-line Joe like myself, find ourselves unable to answer that question. The result? Nobody takes responsibility for the fragile elderly.

Are we afraid to grapple with decisions about a big group of people because we might include or exclude the wrong ones? Something is causing everyone in the system to limit their responsibility when dealing with the average mildly demented, slow-moving ninety-year-old. What's going on here?

At the end of the work day, many primary care doctors leave messages on our voice mail for callers to call 911 or the emergency room. When you call, the office answering machine tells you to call 911 or go to the emergency room if you have problems between 5 PM and 9 AM; anybody with an identifiable illness gets referred to a specialist, and whenever anything changes they go right back to that specialist; when somebody's health gets worse, or when somebody dies, it's a failure of proper medical care. This kind of doctor provides a perfectly adequate service for his young and middle-aged patients but amounts to part of the problem when in charge of primary care for the kind of people I see at home.

Communication between a family doctor and people who organize and provide home support is sometimes not very good. Problems occur in both directions. Doctors may feel awkward working with people trained only to do personal care. A home support agency may have a fragile elderly person who is in crisis and worry that there may be a medical cause for the crisis and that they are not trained to find it. There can be a conflict here, too, if the home support is having problems because of their funding or their personnel or if their program mandate isn't quite sufficient to care for an old person whose needs have suddenly increased. The family doctor may be saying, as I have many times, that the elderly person's problems are being investigated, everything medical that can reasonably be done is being done, and that what we need is more care. The agency may be tempted, at this point, to insist on hospital admission because it is the gold-standard answer to medical questions but also because it effectively ends their responsibility for care at home.

For people responsible in the community, when dependence accelerates in an elderly person and resources are therefore inadequate, the solution seems obvious by simple default. It isn't as though there are dozens of alternatives. If we can't deal with her, she goes to the hospital. Never mind what the doctor says.

The wonderful, kindly, day-to-day nurses, home support workers, and other people who work directly with old people at home don't want to be responsible for not having done enough medically. It isn't a home support worker's or a nurse's responsibility to decide whether someone is having a heart attack or has cancer, and if so, whether it's reasonable to try to treat it. That argument, in my experience, often comes up when the home support we have to offer just isn't enough to meet an old person's often temporary needs.

And at the other, high-tech end of the spectrum of care are the emergency rooms, hospitals, and specialists who may receive a fragile old person, often sent by in-home care providers who are at their wits' end (I imagine these folks' sigh of relief when instead of getting the doctor herself on the telephone, they hear the medical office assistant's recorded voice telling them to go to the emergency room). These capable, highly trained hospital doctors tell us the names of seven things the matter with the old gentleman (all of which somebody already knew about; none of which anybody can do anything about), and offer admission to hospital, more referrals, and more investigations. For them the responsibility is technical and disease focused, as it should be. The idea of assuming responsibility for what's actually going to happen to a ninety-year-old whose problems they know perfectly well they can't fix just isn't in their informal job description. That job description consists of the antithesis of dying: its prevention and rescue from it. So taking responsibility for unsolvable problems really, properly, *isn't* part of what people involved in critical care ought to be doing. Nobody is asking me to do brain surgery; nobody should ask a brain surgeon to do good primary care.

Friends and families just feel overwhelmed. Like the home care agencies whose policies and procedures don't allow for unanswered questions or prompt provision of more support, sons, daughters, spouses, and neighbors feel in no position to make the fatal pronouncement that Dad Just Needs to Be Kept Comfortable. Time after time I hear from families that what they were told at the hospital didn't make sense, didn't explain what was going on, and didn't include any advice about what to do. Again, the busy hospital doctors have done their job. But it is a rare, very confident, determined, and usually well-qualified family member who takes this big scary bull by the horns without advice.

You can see how it happens regularly that nobody is prepared to face the usual course of a frail elderly person's likely future, call it what it is, and do the necessary things to make it tolerable.

So the medical system as the fragile elderly receive it is populated with shrugged shoulders and turned backs. Nothing professionally incorrect or even inhumane here: after the most careful evaluation and often with a very sincere explanation, the conclusion is "not my responsibility." Nobody's responsibility. Not home care agencies and nurses, not hospital doctors or specialists, not families, and not most of us in primary care. And as I said, there are some pretty good reasons for this situation. How can anybody take responsibility for problems nobody can solve? Is it fair to ask professional people to make decisions all the time about a future that, however short-term and generally bleak it may seem, is impossible to predict?

Mrs. Seppanen is an example of someone nobody took responsibility for. She didn't need any of the specialists she saw, and, although she needed and received daily help with cleaning, taking a bath, and meal preparation toward the end of her life, she found her most important needs—her *interests*, really—opposed by the professionals in the community who were there to see to them. The nephew cared about her but would happily have seen her in a nursing home. Case managers and mental health workers found her increasingly impossible to deal with, imagining, I'm sure, the next disaster and how they would justify not having seen to her safety. I have sympathy with this because I've been confronted with it so many times myself. She was demented and so of course was going to have completely impractical and unreasonable demands. But staying and dying in her home were needs that preceded and outranked the dementia, because from Mrs. Seppanen's point of view being in her home was the reason for her being in the world.

Knowing this and having trouble convincing anybody of it, I found it difficult working to meet her medical needs when everybody else seemed determined to limit their exposure to risk. Thus, I had a fight on my hands with every crisis. Keeping the house clean, taking her pills, changing the dressings on her legs, keeping safe from burglars, even getting enough to eat were secondary to Mrs. Seppanen. Her *value*, as we might call it, was *herself in her home*. And there was absolutely nobody willing to be responsible, to take the risk, of giving that to her. Her happy ending was just good luck. Nine times out of ten it doesn't work out that way.

In the last chapter I talked about how the hospital, misapplied to the problems of elderly patients, looks like a maze that leads inexorably toward its own center. The only way out may be feet first. But there is a strange and fascinating flip side to this usual scenario, and it is as clear and horrifying an example of abandonment of responsibility as any. Fragile elderly people who don't escape the hospital maze by dying eventually get discharged. Mary McCarthy, for example. I'm not the first person to notice what some of the language involved in hospital care reveals. "Discharge" is exactly what happens, and that word is like a haiku description of the process. Pull the trigger. Over the side. The whole time the hospital machinery is grinding away on the elderly person's list of problems, that obsessive need to manage every risk perfectly is being quietly opposed by another reality: "We need the bed!" At some point, presuming some exhaustion of the risk-managing hospital machinery, and the person's survival, the seesaw tips. This usually happens, for some reason, around 9:30 in the morning. And it's fifteen or twenty minutes later that a family member gets a phone call to come and get his mother or father.

Next, the same kind of almost military disregard for anything but the hospital's overriding needs, that grin-and-bear-it approach to priorities we see played out in the ambulance, in the emergency room, and on the hospital wards, results in one of the most dramatic gaps in health care. There are people in the hospital responsible for discharge planning, but discharge, no matter how much planning goes into it, in my experience virtually never plays out the way it's supposed to.

The scenario might go like this: "Um, your mother is ready to go home," says the voice on the telephone. "But I just talked to the doctor yesterday, and he said it would be at least two more weeks." "Discharge date is today, and discharge time is noon." "But what about looking after her at home?" "Don't worry, that's all been taken care of." "What about her medication?" "There'll be a prescription." "How does she get home?" "An ambulance is waiting." "But she can't get from her bed to the bathroom." "A home care occupational therapist will visit and take care of all that." Et cetera.

The community doctor does not know about the discharge, does not know what the discharge medications are, and has no idea what happened in the hospital, never having been consulted by the hospital doctors, but is expected to seamlessly carry on with everything that's been, however ill-advisedly, done. More important, the patient experiences a breathtaking drop, of which the doctor's scrambling to get up to speed is only a small part.

To continue to describe the usual hospital discharge scenario, to which there are exceptions, looking after your mother at home *hasn't* all been taken care of. The home support agency gets an e-mail Monday about a discharge last Friday and gets around to its assessment in three or four days. The discharge prescription never coincides with the medication listed, assuming anything is listed, on the discharge summary, which the family doctor receives a copy of three to five weeks later, if ever. What is she supposed to be taking? (Never mind the wrongness of whatever medication regimen somebody, or some group of people, intended her to take.) A second-year medical resident on his first day of service has been told to write the discharge prescription, and he does the best he can between illegible hospital orders and a completely indecipherable computer printout in the file. He makes mistakes. He's in a hurry because there's an elderly person in emergency with diarrhea, he's had two calls from the ward because old people have called out or fallen out of bed, and he's due at rounds to hear a presentation on treating high blood pressure in the elderly. The family physician doesn't even know for certain the details of the bad medicine he will need to discontinue.

The walker, commode, bedpan, catheter supplies, weight-distributing mattress, and all the other things imagined by hospital physiotherapists, social workers, and nurses just aren't there. For sure, many of them are either unnecessary or necessary only because of events in the hospital that were themselves completely unnecessary, but somehow it would help everyone to have a sense that the elderly person's needs *mattered*, if there were some practical attention paid to even a completely impractical attempt to meet them. Confronting Mary McCarthy as I did at the beginning of this book is a very familiar experience, and not just because she was in bad, and worse, shape or just because she was on a lot of dangerous medicine. The way I find her is also the result of the breathtaking drop from the hospital to the rest of the world. By the time she hits the ground, the hospital has already turned its attention (washing its hands, of course, several times a day) to its daily priorities.

I had a conversation recently with an academic geriatric doctor responsible for programs and administration in our community. She was filled with enthusiasm for all sorts of in-hospital solutions to the problems elderly people face. I waited until she was finished and then tried to impress on her that I thought the solution wasn't in the hospital but in the community, where we have a chance to keep elderly people out of the hospital in the first place. She looked at me as if I were speaking a foreign language. Surely, though, if her approach to crisis in the elderly never completely goes away, and if in spite of the apparent insanity of it, we keep right on putting old people in the hospital, we will find a way to start letting them out of there gently. Reasonably. Won't we?

Henri Boisvert is my other chosen model for what happens when old people fall between the cracks. How charming he is, posing for us (I don't think I mentioned that he usually expresses his fear of women not by cowering under the bedsheets but by shrieking the most unbelievable obscenities whenever a small, quiet female nurse's aide student, for example, comes into the room). Henri's situation is an example of something I see quite a bit, though I used to see it much more often when I worked regularly in nursing homes or long-term-care facilities. This is just bad care. Malpractice, a lawyer might call it. But in the same way that doctors sincerely and correctly practicing prevention can cause preventable disasters, nobody necessarily shows up as negligent when we try to analyze why Henri nearly died. Bad care doesn't always require bad doctoring, unless we redefine "doctoring" to include taking that very responsibility that nobody wants. Bad care is, in this situation, nobody watching the big picture, so the patient got fragmented care. He fell between the cracks.

Henri Boisvert's fragmented-care story involved a bit more than just the hands-off, hot-potato approach. It's another example of a medical system designed for a completely different type of person with completely different needs than his. There exist in my profession unwritten rules, customs, and tolerances we live by, which work perfectly well as long as a patient can advocate for himself and evaluate service like any other reasonable consumer. These can drop demented old people like Henri into a void.

In a hospital, or when one is treating someone capable of following directions, the way doctors do business is usually workable. Doctors tend to be on call for one another outside of office hours, and they have a loose set of rules about communication related to this shared responsibility. One doctor may presume, for example, that his treatment of someone's back pain by telephone will be communicated to the original doctor by the patient, if necessary. Another doctor may respond to a call from a nurse at the hospital by prescribing for another physician's patient based on the nurse's report and assume that his colleague will see on Monday morning what he did and make any necessary adjustments. Yet another doctor might respond to an out-of-office-hours call by suggesting no action at all when he realizes that the patient has recently been seen by a specialist and some investigations are still pending. All these things are sensible and safe unless the hospital involved is actually a nursing home and the patient is someone who can't speak for himself.

With that in mind let's take a more detailed look at what happened to Henri Boisvert. One of the toughest problems in primary care geriatrics is agitated, noisy, combative, troubled people with dementia. They are found most often in nursing homes, but they can also be found at home and most definitely in hospitals. They are a problem that nobody enjoys dealing with, partly because it's just plain difficult, and partly because dealing with it means constantly reevaluating the consequences of trial and error. Treatment is always tentative and subject to careful follow-up.

Dementia causes people to lose their ability to think and remember. As it gets worse, it must be terrifying for the demented
person always to live in a state of bewilderment. I imagine this
being like every minute just having woken up in a completely
strange, sometimes scary place and having no idea what's going
on. No wonder memory-impaired people shout for help, make
loud, repetitive demands, bang and throw objects, try to hit caregivers, bite, rummage at random in other people's belongings,
and pace back and forth until they are exhausted.

Articles on what to do about that kind of behavior in dementia always tell us to be sure that the person isn't shouting or
running around because of something we can fix: a pain, being
sick in some way, or just being afraid of something specific. But
when an elderly person gets upset and starts yelling, the whole
floor of a nursing home can be affected, so something has to be
done quickly. It just isn't always possible to do the kind of careful investigation to find treatable causes that everybody knows
should be done *before* starting some kind of calming medication
that quiets the person temporarily and gets everybody back to a
livable situation.

The trouble with Mr. Boisvert wasn't just that he was a long-
standing agitated screamer. That particular nursing facility had
another problem that is very common: not enough family doctors. Henri had had three or four of them over the past couple
of years, but through bad luck all of them had quit the nursing
home, moved away, or retired. In the few months before I saw
him, *nobody* was doing his primary care. It fell to the doctor on
call for the nursing unit.

I have always hated being on call. Part of why it's so difficult
is that health problems don't respect office hours. This is true at

every level: in hospitals where somebody might need an operation quickly, an anesthiologist must be available, and so must a
surgeon and, depending on the sophistication of the hospital, a
kidney specialist, a plastic surgeon, or a neurologist. When you
are the person who might have to respond quickly, you have to
be available, which includes being able to assume a businesslike
frame of mind and being within beeper range. And the beeper always goes off at the wrong moment.

Among specialists the job to be done is often something well-
known and understood because of your training and experience:
this twelve-year-old needs her appendix out, this facial fracture
needs repair, this schizophrenic needs to be treated and pro-
tected. I don't mean to suggest for a moment that it's simple or
easy, but most often it's *defined*. The rigidity of the hospital setting has its advantages at times. At least you can usually get some
of the information you need to do your job properly. In primary
care, especially with fragile elderly people, the situation a doctor gets called into may have nuances, sensitivities, advance directives, and treatments that have already been tried, which you
need to know about. And if it's the weekend or late at night, if the
person is at home or in a nursing home, that information may be
hard to come by—illegible, just absent, or simply unknown to a
replacement nurse unfamiliar with the patient.

So what happens? On-call doctors are only human and are
likely to ask themselves: Do I have to go and see this person?
Do I have to review the chart? Is this problem dangerous, and if
so, could I fix it? And they give themselves the answers to those
questions not in a perfect Platonic vacuum but in consideration
of how far they have to go, how tired they are, whether they've
just left home for an outing, and so on. They will also decide, in
the same way, on what a safe and reasonable strategy would be to

carry the situation over until a primarily responsible doctor can do the proper thing: be sure (in the case of an agitated, noisy, demented person) that the patient isn't shouting or running around because of something that can be fixed.

When Henri Boisvert's shouting got really bad at different times (and it was getting slowly worse), the nurse would contact the doctor on call, describe the behavior, give whatever background information he was able to provide, and ask for help. Because the doctor on call understands that the behavior has to be controlled independent of its cause, sedative medication was prescribed. Because the doctor on call at night or on the weekend assumes that there is a primary care colleague responsible, and because "rounding up the usual suspects" to make sure there is no easily treatable cause for the behavior requires a full examination, blood tests, and possibly x-rays, which can't easily be done outside daytime hours, the sedative may be all the doctor on call does. She might phone and leave a message for the responsible primary doctor, or she might not.

So we can understand how screaming Henri got medication and no proper diagnostic workup: there didn't happen to be anybody doing his primary care. Nobody was responsible.

The head nurse saw herself as responsible, of course, but not directly responsible for *medical* care. The patient's screaming calmed down with the sedative prescribed by phone, and she properly assumed the on-call doctor had done the right thing. Two weeks later, when Henri was shouting loudly again on the weekend because in some way his brain had overcome the first effect of the sedative medication, that responsible nurse was concerned enough on Monday (even though Henri was quiet again from a dose increase provided by another doctor on call) to request a visit from a psychiatrist.

The psychiatry specialist came in, reviewed the chart, looked at the existing medication, examined Mr. Boisvert from a psychological perspective, and made the diagnosis of "psychological and behavioral symptoms of dementia." In his consultation letter he recommended some tests to be sure there was no underlying physical problem and suggested a medical evaluation. He started antidementia medicine. Some tests came back normal.

The third time an on-call doctor was paged outside regular hours, that third doctor understood that the patient had been seen by a psychiatrist and antidementia medicine had been started, and he decided what was needed was behavior control while waiting for the medication to work. More sedation. This third doctor was reassured that a psychiatrist had seen, recently examined, and treated the patient.

Nobody was thinking about prevention or rescue here. This near-disaster was the result of fragmented care and of nobody taking responsibility. Especially responsibility for this most troublesome and least attractive kind of old person. But I think the most dangerous ingredient in the stew the system cooked up for Henri Boisvert was a kind of false reassurance that as long as a patient is in an institution, the policies and procedures of the institution are met, someone calls the doctor, and a specialist has been involved, everything is okay. Nobody did anything really *wrong* here. The near-deadly scene developed just because nobody was looking at the whole movie—the big picture. That, as I've said before, is a failure of primary care.

It's the family doctor's job to understand everything remotely relevant to an old person's care and life, take it all into account, and make decisions (or help with them) accordingly. When nobody is doing that, or if a primary care doctor sees herself as a kind of referral clearinghouse, the safety switch is off and old people get hurt.

I'd better say that I chose Henri Boisvert as an example because I'm familiar with him, not to tell you about my own success. I was the new broom there, as it happened, but I could just as easily have been any of the perfectly capable people on call, unintentionally making things worse, as I fear I've done dozens of times without even knowing it.

We need to have a radical change in the way we think about doing our jobs in health care. A family doctor visiting fragile old people at home and available to bring commonsense medical care to them whenever necessary is part of the solution. But only part. A completely different understanding of these people's needs is necessary if we're going to stop trying to help them with drugs and hospitals and keep them from falling between the cracks.

But the fragile elderly are not the only victims of the lack of fit between them and the medical system. In a serious traffic accident involving two vehicles normally neither vehicle avoids damage. And they both contain drivers and passengers. Real people who were moments ago just travelling along a road are suddenly in terrible trouble, or dead. Chapter 7 deals with the other vehicle: the medical care system.

# 7 You Should See the Other Guy
## The System in Trouble

### JENNIFER CHOW

Jennifer Chow was a thirty-year veteran in the medical system. Trained as a nurse, she later studied administration for two years and then took a job with a big-city hospital, working her way up to a junior vice presidency with responsibility for bed allocation. She consulted privately outside her day job. She was working on her PhD.

Jennifer got a phone call at 9 PM on Friday, when she thought she was safely home and out of the fray. It was Doug Peters, on duty in the emergency room. They had just turned away two ambulances, one with a seriously sick child, the other headed in from a highway accident. He was sure they had been diverted to the fairly close other hospital in town, but he didn't know the status over there. The ER was overflowing. Every available stretcher was full, and so were all the hallways; some of the people had been there for three days. It was a particularly busy night.

When Jennifer downloaded her computer stats for the past twenty-four hours, the average age of people in the six-hundred-bed hospital was seventy-four; on the medical wards it was eighty.

Lengths of stay were high in spite of changes made to the numbers by removing people who were still in hospital simply because they had nowhere to go.

Jennifer got on the phone to the first of her nurse managers to see how many people she could discharge. She was not optimistic. You can't send chronically sick old people who are unable to manage for themselves home without some kind of support, and for most of the ones awaiting discharge home support was a problem.

Meanwhile on Second West, a general internal-medicine ward, the daughter, son-in-law, and two grandchildren of Dorothy Higgins had come to visit. Dorothy, aged eighty-eight, had been admitted three weeks previously with a sudden, very severe pain in the middle of her back. She had suffered a partial collapse of a vertebra, and the emergency room doctor didn't think the pain could be controlled at home. Her family physician heard of the admission two days later and tried to discharge her so that he could care for her at home, but the internist in charge of the ward was concerned because Dorothy had some abnormalities in her blood oxygen and an unexplained impairment of kidney function. She also appeared to be short of breath, a condition that was under investigation.

During the investigation she had an elevated white blood cell count, which a resident trainee specialist attributed to infection, and she was started on antibiotics. Three days later diarrhea developed, and an IV had to be started because of dehydration. Unable to get out of bed, Dorothy couldn't get to the bathroom, so a catheter was inserted in her bladder. The family noticed during the second week that she was beginning to be a little confused. Nobody foresaw discharge from the hospital any time soon.

THE WRONG FIT between fragile elderly and the medical system hurts the system as well as the elderly. The story I'm telling does not have a good guy versus bad guy plot. Instead, complicated and morally ambiguous characters just get into trouble with one another.

As your children grow up, you get to see how TV programming for various age groups has evolved since you were young yourself. My conclusion in general is that it's much, much worse. But one Saturday several years ago I stopped behind the chair where my fifteen-year-old son was watching a sort of daredevil documentary. I had just come back from the hospital, where I had spent two hours in an unsuccessful struggle to discharge a lady very much like Dorothy Higgins back to her home. The documentary TV show grabbed my attention for a reason that I couldn't see at first but that later gradually dawned on me.

A million-dollar Ferrari racing car was being used to pull an ordinary loaded freight train. A young announcer shouted at the camera with increasing excitement; this was all about speed versus power. The racing-car driver in his special suit and helmet climbed into the Formula 1 machine, started the engine, and put the car in gear. The huge flat black rear tires spun on the railroad ties, spitting up gravel and pouring forth blue smoke. We could hear rocks clanging off the metal on the front of the first boxcar. The racing engine screamed, and the camera showed tremendous tension on the cable connecting the car to the train. The train creaked but didn't budge.

After a few minutes a blast of smoke and oil came from under the hood of the car. Technicians rushed with their stainless-steel equipment to replace the burnt-out engine, which they accomplished in only a minute or two. The car started up again, and the whole thing was repeated.

Eventually I realized I was watching something oddly familiar. I had just come from an attempt to prevent the hospital from misapplying its extremely sophisticated solutions to one of my old patients, and I was as usual astounded at how bizarrely wrong it was to keep that particular lady, who couldn't possibly benefit from any of the technology there, in the hospital. I saw in this ridiculous TV-show experiment an example of what happens when the task and what we try to do it with don't fit. Nothing wrong with the racing car: it's close to perfect for what it was designed to do. It is incredibly expensive and wonderfully highly specialized. But it burnt out fast (and cost even more) when somebody tried to make it do what it couldn't.

A hospital is a wonderful thing when it is doing the job for which it was designed and, in a relative way, perfected. If it had been physically possible to rescue Martha Cleaver in Chapter 5, I'm sure it would've happened. The professionals' performance filled my doctor's heart with pride. The sophistication of the technology available in a hospital is also impressive. To really understand just how good our medical system can be, however, I think you have to be a patient.

I've been one, fortunately only a couple of times. It's an amazing feeling to sit across the desk from a medical specialist (to whom I've referred quite a few patients) and hear him discuss *my* problems. That he has in front of him state-of-the-art images of my degenerated spine, that he has reviewed the images and agrees with the university radiologist who has also read them, that he has examined me carefully with all his training and experience, and that he looks at me and tells me I don't have multiple sclerosis or cancer provides reassurance on a level that's pretty hard to beat. On the occasion I'm describing here, I left the medical office building singing to myself and skipping on the sidewalk like a six-year-old. Millions of people out there have much less trivial reasons to thank modern health care for its miracles.

Until I had my blinding flash of insight watching the racing car trying to pull the freight train on TV, I had been so preoccupied with the bad effects of the medical system on my patients that I hadn't really stopped to think much about what is happening, and what is probably going to happen, to that medical system itself.

As we try to help very old people with programs, drugs, specialized care, technology, and procedures designed to meet completely different needs, those resources get used up, relatively speaking. When hospital beds, operating rooms, and x-ray and laboratory facilities are occupied by very old people who can't benefit from these resources anyway, those resources will not be available for people who *can* benefit from them, and the needs the resources were first designed to meet don't get met.

It takes months to see medical specialists because their time is occupied evaluating old people's health problems as if they could be fixed using their operations and other treatments. Although it is often argued that wait times are longer in a single-payer system (Canada's, for example) than in one emphasizing private payment (like in the United States, for example), the time it takes to see a specialist or to have a particular operation performed varies tremendously *within* each of these systems. And the continuing argument over private versus public payment suggests that there is no clear-cut answer to which type of system is better with respect to how long one waits for service. But old people's health problems usually can't be fixed by getting to the head of the lineup for a specialist, an operation, or an imaging study.

Drug payment plans are also forced to limit benefits because their budgets are gobbled by expensive, futile, and harmful preventive prescriptions for people for whom the drugs are not demonstrably effective. Emergency-response budgets balloon, or emergency-response efficiency sags, because we have no better response to caregiver burnout than calling an ambulance.

And these resources are needed, make no mistake. At the same time as the fragile elderly population is exploding, the rest of us have problems that the conventional, legitimate high-tech medical system could actually do something about if the resources were not otherwise occupied. This situation is getting worse, not better. And there is lots of information to suggest that it will continue to do so unless we make some fundamental changes to how the system is used.

Information about populations, their health care, and projections into the future do help us to understand the state of the medical system now and down the road. But like all statistics, the information I present here, which I think is interesting and important, is subject to a certain amount of interpretation.

Everyone seems to understand that populations in the Western world will continue to be defined by the post–World War II baby boom for another few decades. Statistical projections of the shape of those populations suggest that they will have an impact on all sorts of things well beyond that. The proportion of people over sixty-five is expected to increase from about 12 percent to about 20 percent by 2050, more than a 50 percent increase. This would be at a time when the baby boomers are starting to hit the age of one hundred. But people over eighty-five, now just under 2 percent of the population, will grow by 135 percent over the same time period, to well over 4 percent. And much of that increase will occur after 2030.

The usual analogy to describe this is the "squaring of the population pyramid." Traditionally, because people are more and more likely to die as they get older, a population diagram that shows how many people there are in different age groups looks like a pyramid—large numbers in the young age groups at the base, and smaller and smaller numbers in the older and older age groups toward the peak. But as the boomers like me age, a population bulge slowly pushes its way up the pyramid like an animal being digested by a snake. The bulge gets smaller with passing time, but eventually it enters the highest age categories, enlarges the traditionally tiny pyramid top, and squares the pyramid shape. But that squaring is not expected to disappear when we boomers die and disappear upward out of the diagram.

This trend has been discussed by health planners, economists, and theorists of resource allocation of every type and has been used to argue for higher taxes, lower taxes, socialized medicine, free-enterprise medicine, more hospitals, fewer hospitals. The brute fact is that we will face—we as a society will in large part be—millions and millions of very elderly people for a significant time in the future. That fact doesn't ever disappear, no matter what use we try to put it to.

That increase in over-eighty-fives has a disproportionate impact on the use of all sorts of health resources. The average number of medical diagnoses per person increases with age. The relatively small proportion of people over eighty-five will therefore account for a very large percentage of all illness. There is debate over what the resulting impact on costs will be, but there is no doubt about the amount of chronic disease we will see among these very elderly people. More than doubling their numbers will mean more than doubling the large proportion of chronic diseases they account for. Imagine for a moment that you are a health-economics planner. All you have to do to end up with numbers nobody wants to hear is start thinking about dealing with every single chronic disease problem in every single very elderly person, as things look in a future scenario you see on your screen. And the more exactly every single one of the chronic disease problems is treated according to its guidelines, the worse the picture gets.

There is not much evidence-based or even published information about the extent of harm to the medical system that comes from misusing it. So, much of the information and conclusions presented here come from my experience. The damage to health care that I see nearly every day in my work with the elderly can be summarized as follows.

First, guidelines-driven prevention results in a monstrous waste of money on drugs that do more harm than good. These days government-funded or privately funded drug plans often provide medication doctors say we need. The exact nature of these plans varies depending on the medical system. But it doesn't make much difference whether a drug plan is funded privately, like private-paid health insurance, or publicly. The amount of money available is simply limited. And the plan must therefore make decisions about what to pay for under what circumstances. Some plans pay for Viagra, for example, and some don't. Some will pay for expensive drugs to treat heartburn only after the cheaper ones have failed.

I spent eight years as a consultant for the government drug-payment agency where I live and sat on the committee that made decisions about which drugs would be covered and which not. Each decision involved not only the effectiveness and safety of the drugs but also their cost. Everyone on the committee knew that the amount of money allocated for drug treatment among the three million or so people covered by the plan was limited. What we didn't discuss very much was the issue of waste. How many useless and harmful prescriptions are written every year? How much preventive treatment is provided to people in whom prevention has no rational basis in any sort of evidence?

Information to answer these questions is hard to come by. Part of the problem is the ambiguous definition of the idea of "waste" where preventive drug treatment is concerned. Drug plans, as we will see in the next chapter, are not in a position to second-guess prescribers when their prescriptions conform to usual preventive guidelines. It's the "evidence" problem again; there is no evidence supporting prevention in fragile old people, but for exactly the same reasons, there is also very limited evidence to support a decision *not* to treat them preventively if a doctor says they should be. This situation is not confined to the drug plan I worked for, of course. It exists everywhere that medication is paid by a "third party." The kind of waste that concerns me is a universal problem.

Raw data on drug expenditures in the United States shows an overall cost of around US$275 billion per year (projected from 2006–07 numbers) and growing. Canada recorded an approximately population-proportional US$27 billion in 2007. The part of this huge expenditure going to preventive medication is increasing, but the true proportion (and the rate of increase) is hidden by the fact that many drugs are used both for treatment and for prevention. My experience in general medical practice suggests that drugs prescribed for prevention may be approximately half of all prescribed drugs. Certainly the proportion would be over one-third.

The next question we must ask, then, is, How much of that very large preventive expenditure is made without supporting evidence? Generally utilized numbers in Western countries set the "elderly" (people over the age of sixty-five) at 10 to 15 percent.

Among them, the "frail" are about 15 to 20 percent. This produces about 2 percent frail elderly within the total population, which is somewhere close to the usually accepted proportion of 3 percent frailty overall. We recognize that these numbers are fraught with problems to do with definition: What's old? What's frail? Whose country are we talking about? But although frail people are only 2 to 3 percent of the population, they are generally understood to consume about 30 percent of the health care dollars. Of course, not all fragile people are elderly, but they are unusual enough that they have little impact on the numbers discussed here.

Based on these somewhat doubtful approximations, and if you accept my idea that prevention in frailty is not supported by evidence, a worrisome dollar number starts to loom. Dozens of billions per year would potentially be involved just in North America.

But another way of looking at wasted resources with preventive drugs is to ask how many treatable conditions go untreated because we can't afford to treat them—*because we're wasting money on useless care.* For six months or so recently I took over a group of twenty people in a "complex care" nursing home as a favor to a friend who moved his practice. During that time I stopped about half the drugs the patients were taking, slowly and carefully, with no bad consequences. The answer to the question about how much more treatment we could afford if we weren't wasting money is, lots! Imagine if your drug plan were able to afford very much more coverage at the same price. That would be the world as it should and could be. The medical system would be directing its preventive and therapeutic efforts where they count.

Ambulances and other resources that are used to rescue elderly people are then not available to attend to industrial accidents and heart attacks, which they are most effective at dealing with. Each time a fragile old person wrongly enters that system, somebody who could benefit from it has to wait.

I have made a distinction between a crisis of function in an old person in my practice and a crisis involving a sudden, dangerous condition that someone might die from. In either situation it is easy to see how the medical system's usual response of rescue is triggered: we have no resources that help us to be reasonable and low-key in our response to a crisis primarily involving function. And we tend to be afraid of realistically admitting to ourselves the probable uselessness of trying to rescue someone very elderly and suddenly in danger. The rescue-oriented system's response is blind to its own wrongness as a way of dealing with the kind of crisis that fragile elderly people present. And so we continue to misuse it.

I want to describe two personal experiences to emphasize how shamefully we waste critical care rescue on what doesn't need doing, and what kind of consequences this can have.

Early in my home care practice I was visiting Hannah De Voord, a ninety-year-old lady who lived with her daughter and son-in-law in a suburban house. Formerly a hide-the-bottle alcoholic, Mrs. De Voord was now demented enough that the daughter had control, and the old lady's drinking days were over. Normally I just visited every few weeks and checked over medication, tried to stay on top of the symptoms of her quite severe heart disease and chronic lung problems, documented the progress of the dementia, and tried to slow down Mrs. De Voord's collapsing mobility.

On this occasion something else had gone wrong. Mrs. De Voord was not at all her normal self, hadn't been out of bed for a day and a half, was more confused than before, and wasn't eating. My usual-suspects roundup focused on her abdomen: it felt hard and was silent when I listened carefully with my stethoscope, and there was definite soreness on the left side. I didn't like her lowish blood pressure and slightly speeded-up heart rate.

I sat the daughter down and explained that I thought something dangerous was wrong in her mum's stomach area. Part of the digestive tract might have ruptured, a blood vessel could be blocked or bleeding, or there could be infection in that area. I recognized this as a serious crisis-in-the-elderly scenario, and I made it clear to the daughter that we had an important decision to make. Mrs. De Voord could stay home and be comfortable, and she might die or might get better. Or, she could go to the hospital, where there was a slim chance that something dangerous could be repaired by surgery. But I knew, because of my patient's lung and heart disease, and because of the probable future of her dementia, that emergency surgery would be very unlikely to save her life if her situation was life threatening. I also knew that every capable critical care doctor and surgeon who encountered her would understand these important facts. Going to the hospital was not likely to save her life, I said to the daughter, but the medical staff would keep her comfortable, and the outcome would be the same as if she stayed in her familiar home.

The daughter thought this over and asked several questions. I sensed through our conversation her completely understandable reluctance not to do everything possible. It reminded me very much of Mrs. Chau's daughter, whom we met in Chapter 5. Like her, this daughter's decision was to send Mum to the hospital.

My conversation with the emergency dispatch operator took a very familiar form. I was arguing, as a qualified physician who knew the patient well and had examined her in the last fifteen minutes, for a nonemergency, quiet transfer to the hospital. I tried to explain that this was for evaluation and that the problem had been going on for over twenty-four hours. But something I said must have triggered one of the dispatcher's criteria. After I saw my next patient only a few blocks away and drove back past Mrs. De Voord's house, there were two fire trucks sitting diagonally on the road, two ambulances with red lights flashing, a police car diverting traffic at the end of the block, and four emergency personnel visible in the yard, with others no doubt inside running cardiograms, starting an IV, calling the emergency room physician on their cell phones, and preparing for a high-speed transfer to the hospital.

A little more recently I dealt with another, very difficult patient, called Delbert Thompson. The difficulty was that Mr. Thompson didn't remember or understand much because of Alzheimer's dementia. His lifelong pattern of demanding and getting his own way, however, had persisted. Whenever I visited Mr. Thompson, we would have an argument. I dreaded these, but it was hard to avoid them because I had to insist on things like taking medication and keeping drinking under control. One of our recurring differences was what to do with a growth on the side of his face. This thing was nearly an inch across and was, I discovered when Mr. Thompson finally let me take a sample of it, a slow-growing skin cancer. We discussed its treatment again and again. Mr. Thompson absolutely would not leave his home for any procedures, consultations, or investigations. I told him it could be removed with a little operation under local anesthetic but that I wasn't comfortable trying to do it in his home. I felt he would probably die of unrelated causes long before the cancer ever gave him any real trouble, but Mr. Thompson wanted it gone and supported his opinion, for example, by asking, "What kind of doctor are you anyway?"

Looking back, I was rash and overconfident in agreeing to take this thing off his cheek at home one afternoon, with the help of a home support worker. At the time it seemed like the only solution. The little operation was more difficult than I expected, and Mr. Thompson bled quite a bit. I ran out of stitching material, although I thought I had tied off all the blood vessels that were bleeding. Eventually I was able to pull the skin together and close up the wound, happy to get out the door and leaving instructions to the home support worker to press on the bandage for fifteen minutes after I was gone.

Less than an hour later the home support worker called me: blood was still oozing out from under the bandage. I drove over and reluctantly cut open my stitching to try to find the bleeder. I couldn't and now really regretting my decision to do this bit of surgery against my better judgment, I packed the wound with sterile gauze, kept pressure on it myself, called the hospital emergency room, described the situation to the doctor there and requested an ambulance.

The ambulance dispatcher said it would be twenty minutes. An hour later, Mr. Thompson was still oozing blood, and I had gone through my supply of gauze and switched to toilet paper. Gruff and determined, Mr. Thompson was putting on a brave show, but he was getting a little drowsy. The home support worker had stayed way past her quitting time, and I said she could go. I called the ambulance dispatch again, this time explaining that although it wasn't an emergency, we were going to have to get him to the hospital pretty soon. No problem, I was told.

After another half hour Mr. Thompson was asleep, but his heart rate was getting rapid, and I was getting worried. I called dispatch again and said I really needed help. When the ambulance crew arrived, it had been two hours since my first call, and my surgical field looked more like a crime scene.

The paramedics found Mr. Thompson's blood pressure quite low, and now we had trouble rousing him. One of them failed to get an intravenous line started, and just as they were transferring my patient to a stretcher, he had what looked like a seizure. There was still a heartbeat when they left for the hospital, but for once I was encouraging a fast emergency transfer.

Delbert Thompson proved to be made of pretty stern stuff: he had a transfusion and expert surgical repair of his wound, perked up, and was back home the next day arguing with everybody. I made myself a solemn promise *never* to try even minor surgery at home again.

Part of the problem here was my bad judgment. But the other part was the fact that even with a doctor calling urgently for help and in the middle of a big city, there were dangerous delays in getting an ambulance. This near disaster is an example of what can happen when urgently needed reserve resources are busy seeing to nonemergencies like Mrs. De Voord.

I hope these two scenarios of emergency response illuminate what causes my sense of disproportion. A bizarrely inappropriate response to an elderly person in crisis diverts necessary emergency-response people and equipment from the car accidents, critical infections, heart attacks in middle-aged people, industrial injuries, and other important and real health care emergencies, including Mr. Thompson, another elderly person who really needed traditional rescue. Thoughtless adherence to rules and refusing to consider exceptional situations stretches our emergency resources until they are too thin on the ground to be effective.

Misuse of the emergency room can also cause problems. At the community hospital where I once worked as a part-time emergency room doctor, there was an important relationship between our emergency evaluation of patients and the resources of that medium-sized hospital in the city. If the intensive care unit was full, we couldn't admit people who needed that service. If there were no beds on the wards, we couldn't admit people at all. On some busy evenings, especially on the weekend, our emergency facility itself was full. Ambulances sometimes had to be diverted elsewhere.

My experience with wrongly managed crisis in the fragile elderly in the ER features what I call the "Friday Night Suitcase Syndrome." For example, one Friday night around 9:15, Harriet Crow, age ninety-one, arrived at the emergency room. The evening had been difficult, and we were getting close to the point of diverting ambulances to other hospitals. Many of the people I had seen in the past few hours had needed urgent care, referral to specialists, and admission to the hospital. There was a little girl who was hoarse and short of breath, a frightened man with chest pain whose cardiogram and blood test were abnormal, a teenager with a very painful-looking abscess on his backside, an older, obviously drunk man who had thrown up blood, and a woman with a sore neck whose car had been rear-ended.

As I was writing up the admission for the man with chest pain, an ambulance crew came through the door wheeling a stretcher containing Harriet. It was raining out, and she had a white towel over her head. Beneath her, on the lower part of the stretcher, was a small black suitcase.

I had never met Mrs. Crow, but before I could see her to find out what was going on, Margaret MacKenzie, my main ER nurse and a trusted friend, pulled me aside and described the family situation. Mrs. Crow lived with her son Arnold, his wife, and their four teenage kids in a big house by the river. Arnold was a famous drinker and frequent flyer in the ER with problems associated with alcohol. His wife struggled to maintain peace and make ends meet within the family, including looking after her difficult mother-in-law, not always with much help.

Harriet Crow had been in our hospital six months before, also on a Friday night, also with her suitcase. She had spent six weeks on the wards and had finally gone back home once Arnold and his wife got back from being away. Mrs. Crow had heart disease, smoker's lungs, arthritis in her knees and hips, an extremely bad back, a history of a couple of strokes, and intermittent diarrhea. She was able to walk around inside the house but had trouble getting out or even getting to the car. When I read over her file sent down from medical records, there were pages and pages of social work notes describing all the trouble her daughter-in-law had looking after her. Getting her back home had been considered a major victory.

Once I had examined Mrs. Crow and determined that yes, she had heart disease, smoker's lungs, arthritis in her knees and hips, an extremely bad back, a history of a couple of strokes, and intermittent diarrhea (but really nothing new that I could find), Margaret phoned Mrs. Crow's home. There was no answer. We kept her in the hallway outside emergency through most of the weekend, she was admitted to a medical bed in the hospital Sunday afternoon, and the social workers took over on Monday.

The story of Dorothy Higgins, in the vignette at the start of this chapter, completes my anecdotes about homebound frail elderly people and the hospital. Not all the wrong admissions are as obviously pointless as Mrs. Crow's. Mrs. De Voord, who was not in a position to benefit from the excitement of her trip to emergency, with the ambulance running four red lights and hitting fifty miles an hour on some through streets, had a mesenteric vascular occlusion, which is a blocked blood vessel supplying a section of bowel. She was seen that night by a general surgeon and evaluated by an internist, and her situation was then discussed with her daughter. As I had imagined, the predicted likelihood of dying from the surgery needed to save her was extremely high because of her heart and lung problems, and eventually it was decided to consider Mrs. De Voord palliative: keep her comfortable and just wait and see what happened. She joined three other elderly ladies on a subacute hospital ward. Two of them had been admitted to the hospital because of confusion, which had partly resolved, but other problems had arisen. The third woman was awaiting placement in a nursing home.

During the first two nights Mrs. De Voord was in the hospital, the emergency room was diverting ambulances because the hospital was full. Mrs. De Voord died quietly six days after admission. Although she was kept physically comfortable, her death was probably advanced a little by sedatives that were needed to settle her bewilderment at being in an unfamiliar place.

Similar stories are played out everywhere there are hospitals and fragile elderly people, day in and day out. The hospital struggles to do things it was never designed for, the people working there sometimes at their wits' end because of short staffing, too few beds, delays in treatment, diverted ambulances, and long waits for care, while poor fragile old people lie bewildered in the beds needed to do the necessary acute care the hospital should be providing and can't.

Sometime after my epiphany about burning out the racing car by trying to pull a train, another transportation analogy occurred to me. I have characterized the confrontation between the fragile elderly and our prevention-and-rescue medical system as a poor fit, but it is also a kind of collision that causes harm to both vehicles involved.

People who study road crashes tell us that the amount of harm to the occupants of any vehicle in an accident depends on a lot of things. But nobody disputes the idea that you're likeliest to walk away from one of these horrible experiences if your vehicle is designed for safety and if it's really big. And in this fanciful car crash, we're inclined to imagine that the massive, incredibly heavily funded, sophisticated, and risk-oriented health care system represents the much bigger vehicle. Compared with your average Dorothy Higgins, Harriet Crow, or Mary McCarthy, it's no contest, right? But when we look back at some of the statistical information I touched on earlier, we see the health care highway and its traffic a little bit differently.

One doesn't have to have a statistics or economics degree to appreciate that what the medical system is dealing with will become worse in the future with Dorothy, Harriet, and Mary writ large, similar to the huge weight of a loaded freight train. The impact of millions of very old, multiply pathological people has a different character and different effect from any of the fragile little old ladies alone. Modern medical care, with its expensive technology, highly trained professionals, large specialized facilities, and eventually finite drug treatment budgets, is *vulnerable*. The big, dangerous vehicle in this accident may not be Medicare or the university hospital. What the health care system is already suffering, and will suffer in the future, is proportional to the size of what's coming down the road at it: an awful lot of old people. What's coming is huge, getting bigger all the time, and actually already here.

In the early 1980s, when I first got involved in care of the elderly, there was already all sorts of discussion about how we would cope with the coming population explosion among the very old. I remember being at a conference and being shown a cartoon with a couple of easygoing cowboys behind a campfire at the near end of a steep-walled canyon, one strumming his guitar. The caption was, "Oh give me a home where the buffalo roam." In the background, completely filling the canyon from side to side, was an approaching stampede of hundreds of buffalo.

We have known about the coming collision between the fragile elderly and business as usual in medical care for decades. *It's been going on for decades.* Working in the system and watching how we fail to plan for the future, at times I almost feel as if this metaphorical vehicle crash were happening in a terribly bad dream, in monstrously extreme slow motion. The crumpling fenders and flying windshield fragments are today only a millimeter or two removed from when we looked at them in horror six months ago. The damage that is occurring, and that may occur in the future, is terrible and just keeps on happening. Everyone has experienced the kind of dream where you must run but can't. It's as though part of the dream of this hideously slow, destructive accident going on in medical care is that we observers, whether standing on the side of the road or caught in one of the vehicles, are also frozen in the middle of the same kind of slow helplessness. A deadly accident is in progress, and we can't make it stop.

Ambulances called to take old people to the hospital because the family can't cope anymore, emergency room stretchers occupied by unwell old people whose sudden health changes could have been properly handled at home, specialist appointments taken up prescribing pointless, dangerous preventive treatment to people whose doctors misunderstand priorities, imaging studies done to document diseases that nobody would ever dream of treating, and hospital beds occupied for weeks and weeks because guidelines don't permit an end to an otherwise pointless hospital admission are examples of bad health care. And this situation is bad for every one of us, not just the old people pointlessly dragged in misery through it at the end of their lives. If the resources are used up in this way, they simply won't be there to accomplish the things we really need them for.

As long as we who work in the medical system and use it continue to misunderstand what crisis in a homebound old person means, we will persist in helping the system to shoot itself in the foot over and over and over again. We will keep on trying to fix some poor old lady's not being able to get to the bathroom by putting her in a $1,200-a-day hospital bed with iron side rails. We will continue to rush dying people whom we almost certainly can't save (and who, most of the time, don't want to be "saved") into an already overcrowded emergency room where they experience, among their final life events, our desperation at being overwhelmed.

Although there are differences among medical systems in various countries or even regions of countries, this experience of frustration will be familiar to anybody who has seen the collision of fragile old people with the medical system. Everything I have tried and have seen tried seems somehow to underestimate how very focused and vulnerable the medical system is and how very different the needs of the fragile elderly are from those the system can meet.

I have sat on hospital committees and endlessly debated how to move elderly people through the hospital more quickly.

Everyone around the table understands perfectly well that the solution—keeping these people away from the hospital in the first place—is beyond the influence of the hospital. I have listened to and read about global master plans to reorganize health care regions and health authorities of all kinds. An initiative in my province to mobilize the huge and expensive resources of a government health care agency responsible for three million people promised to move health care "closer to home," for example, and the result after ten years is a reshuffling of hardworking bureaucrats and no change whatsoever in care of the elderly in the community. I have written, and been paid over $10,000 for, a several-hundred-page report recommending to that same health care agency coordinated care of the frail elderly at home. As nearly as I can determine, nobody ever read the report.

I have seen several smaller regional so-named innovative programs designed to look after old people at home, none of which involves physicians, provides any twenty-four-hour service (except through the emergency room), or properly supports old people in temporary crisis. I have been involved in the start-up of no fewer than four potential government-funded programs to provide genuinely comprehensive care and support for old people at home, and every one of them has collapsed. I attended a government-sponsored conference three or four years ago designed to gather leaders together, which ended with recommendations for better and more flexible care at home: nothing of the kind has since happened.

For fifteen years or so I have given impassioned presentations to audiences of doctors, health administrators, nurses, and others, singing the same kind of song you hear in this book. Lately, several rural communities near where I live have asked me to give what I think are referred to as inspirational talks on what we need to do to manage my patient population properly. It's too soon to tell what the result of *that* will be, but if past performance is any indication, I am not very optimistic.

To be fair, and in the interest of balance, I have to point out that some home health care programs have succeeded, although modestly. PACE (Program of All-inclusive Care of the Elderly) has developed over thirty-five years in the United States and is still functioning. In the 1970s a very creative group founded On Lok Lifeways, a home care program in the Chinese community in San Francisco. In the late 1980s I visited the program, toured their facilities, and talked to many of the wonderful people working there. PACE has since developed some thirty-seven sites throughout the United States. Many of the programs thrive, and there is a wealth of research and training associated with them. In Canada three or four similar programs exist in various cities.

Unfortunately, these programs have not had a large-scale effect. PACE serves fourteen thousand people. A conservative estimate of the number of frail elderly in the United States in the year 2000 was 9 million, projected to rise to over 12 million by 2020. PACE, the largest program of its kind in the United States, is succeeding at helping less than 0.2 percent of the population theoretically in need!

Why have PACE and other, similar programs not caught on? I don't think anyone knows. But I believe there is resistance to commonsense home care for two general reasons. First, professional, commercial, and otherwise conservative interests in the medical system may foresee loss of control, revenue, and, simply put, *order* if huge numbers of people and those caring for them strike out on their own. But more important, I'm afraid, is our own individual reluctance to abandon what we see as the reliability of the cookbook approach to care.

In spite of real bright spots in the battle to rescue the medical system from its own mistakes, we have not made a lot of progress. Recently I saw another op-ed spread in the newspaper with pictures of a bright young family physician looking after a happy elderly patient. The administrative people responsible for the local system have a new plan for dealing with the coming aging boomers. Primary care! The article gave the impression that this solution to care of the elderly was some sort of new idea. I dug out my scrapbook and there, a little on the yellow side, was a newspaper article from over a decade ago, with a big picture of a serious family doctor taking an old man's blood pressure. Home visits, announced the journalist. The answer to the coming burden of care of the elderly. That serious doctor in the picture ten years ago was me.

The fragile elderly are not getting what they need. Our wrong-headed response to those needs is making their problems worse, not better. And yes, we are also burning out the best of the medical system by insisting on that response. Who is to blame? I have no shortage of answers to that question, and we will take a look at some of them in Chapter 8.

# 8  Lock Them Up and Throw Away the Key
The Villains of the Piece

Thirty years ago the head of one of the world's best-known
drug companies made some remarkably candid comments.
Close to retirement at the time, Merck's gruff and aggressive
chief executive Henry Gadsen spoke to *Fortune* magazine
about his distress that Merck's potential market had been
limited to sick people. Suggesting he would like Merck to be
more like chewing gum maker Wrigley's, Gadsen said it had
long been his dream to make drugs for healthy people, so
Merck would be able to "sell to everyone."

RAY MOYNIHAN AND ALAN CASSELS IN *SELLING SICKNESS*

With the transformation of the doctor from an artisan exercising a skill on personally known individuals into a
technician applying scientific rules to classes of patients,
malpractice acquired an anonymous, almost respectable
status. What had formerly been considered an abuse of confidence and a moral fault can now be rationalized into the

occasional breakdown of equipment and operators. In a complex technological hospital, negligence becomes "random human error" or "system breakdown," callousness becomes "scientific detachment," and incompetence becomes "a lack of specialized equipment."

IVAN ILLICH IN *MEDICAL NEMESIS*

BY NOW YOU understand that I believe a dangerously rigid way of doing health care has evolved and that frail older people are routinely suffering as a result. Who caused this obviously bad situation? If people are being harmed because we practice an oversimplified care that ignores their needs, how did it happen? Is some obscure party encouraging us to stifle the educated instincts of good, experienced professional people in favor of an idiotic consistency?

I have described a medical system that emphasizes prevention and rescue and, in being scientific, at times abandons important priorities like kindness, meeting patients' needs, and common sense. Fragile older people simply don't get the kind of attention they need because nobody in the scientific system we live with is in a position to understand, let alone meet, their needs. But scientific health care includes some frankly wonderful things. Anyone unhappy with the way we do business, and trying to figure out how to improve things, has to acknowledge that in many ways and for many other people modern medical care is very good indeed. It just doesn't work for the fragile elderly.

If I'm even partly correct in believing that people like my patients suffer more than everybody else from rigid and oversimplified modern ways of doing business in health care, and the health care system is groaning under the burden of inflicting all this misery, don't we have to try to do something about it? But how are we supposed to go about that?

First let's look at three or four of the most popular targets for blame. Over and over again I see angry fingers pointed at the same nasty old perpetrators: the drug industry, academic doctors, doctors in general, and health care administration in all its forms. They all tend to be viewed dimly when any failing of health care is being considered. In discussing each of these usually blamed groups of people I am reporting the common wisdom, not a view that I myself subscribe to. The picture is nowhere near as simple as those who think we can focus blame for bad health care imagine it to be. But let's take a look at each group and see what we think.

I've mentioned that for about eight years I had a part-time job with the drug payment agency where I live. As its medical consultant I sat on the Drug Benefit Committee and helped with its decisions about what drugs we would buy for the people in our region. This drug payment agency is similar in many ways to other third-party payers in a privately funded system like that in the United States. Because the decisions of the committee I sat on potentially had an impact on drug sales, locally at least, all during those years I pointedly avoided communication with anybody from the drug industry because conversations with them could have led to conflict of interest.

But before those years I had more or less the same relationship with drug industry sales or "detail" people that most doctors in my community (and all over the world) have. I might have been a little more skeptical than some, but I attended my share of drug company lunches and dinners, hockey games, and weekends at local resorts, courtesy of whichever drug company salesperson happened to have some promotional money to spend.

Drug companies regularly paid me to give talks to groups of doctors they had lured into the room through gifts. I say regularly, but getting paid to speak at a drug company event was infrequent for me because the kind of talk I'm qualified to give rarely involved any kind of drug treatment. Specialists I know whose work involves mainly drug treatment of common conditions speak much more often, sometimes at distant and desirable locations, and sometimes for a pretty high price.

I also helped organize medical education for other doctors, so I often used to phone up drug industry representatives to ask for money for our education sessions. Medical education events were one source of revenue for our local doctors' organization, and so we would always try to get as much funding up front as we could to help keep the association alive. The usual deal was that we would ask various drug companies for a few thousand dollars here, a few thousand dollars there, and in return we would provide for them a table in the lobby of our conference, where they could display their wares to the captive audience of a hundred or more prescribing physicians.

Now many people—possibly you among them—get upset about the sleaziness they see in this kind of arrangement, but it may not be quite as bad as it looks. Gullible and unsophisticated though we doctors are, most of us have a pretty fair idea of when the butter is being applied to the bread and somebody is trying to influence our prescribing habits. And so at the coffee break of a typical medical education conference, you'll see doctors wandering around the lobby, chatting with drug representatives and listening to their pitch but not impressed by the extremely one-sided "evidence" these good folks present for the superiority of the products they are selling.

I don't think that the little story I want to relate here could happen today. This was at least twelve years ago, when the rules governing drug industry corporate behavior in most countries weren't quite as well defined as they are now. But it will give you a taste of the kind of cookies the drug industry bakes or would like to bake.

At the end of a long afternoon two industry salespeople were sitting in my office for our second meeting. At our first meeting I had requested a $5,000 grant for the course coming up, with the usual promotional opportunity offered. I was expecting, and hoping for, an offer of about $2,500 from them. Everyone has a job to do, and these two lovely people have no doubt long since moved on in their careers. But to characterize them that afternoon as *slick* would be a big understatement. Both (a man and a woman) were attractive young people in their midtwenties, dressed like junior tax lawyers and smelling like Chanel. Their hair though perfectly in place, looked wet, apparently to give you the idea that they had both just come from a workout. They were very courteous.

"So, how did you make out getting the grant for us?" I asked. "Doctor," said the man, "We'd like to give you five thousand dollars. But we would *love* to give you ten thousand dollars."

"Ten thousand dollars?" I managed (I could picture how impressed the other association doctors were going to be). Yes, they both reassured me, they were authorized to provide that much money. But there was a catch. Did I think it would be, or could be, in any way possible for one of our speakers to mention [the brand name of a new and expensive antibiotic]?

I was a bit stunned. I told them I would think it over and get back to them. As soon as they left, I picked up the phone and called my friend who was going to give the talk on infectious diseases. I asked him whether he thought he would be mentioning the particular product in question. Although I didn't tell him what was going on, he probably had an idea. He offered to check with his subspecialist colleague and the published guidelines and call me back. Finally, yes, he was able to mention the product in good conscience. He said he would have mentioned it anyway. We had a very successful course that year.

The big corporations that produce drugs today are very much involved in modern medical care, way beyond just producing and marketing the pills themselves. They now pay for and do most drug trials. Of course they promote medication. They pay for advocacy groups for people with specific diseases and have for decades paid for and organized all sorts of continuing education for doctors, through the kind of thing I described with our doctors' organization, from paying speakers to bringing hundreds of physicians to expensive resorts at exotic locations, down to giving specialist-trainee resident doctors in hospitals free pens and doughnuts. This is simply promoting one's product.

Industry's influence on medical practice has certainly been discussed before. There is a strong and vocal movement among academic doctors and regulatory agencies to prevent undue influence. There is lots and lots of popular and academic information on this subject, and fundamentalists exist on both sides of the issue. If you want a beautifully readable introduction to the anti-industry side of the subject, *Selling Sickness* by Alan Cassels and Ray Moynihan (quoted at the beginning of this chapter) would get you started. I am not going to review this continuing controversy in depth here, but it is reasonable to ask whether there might be a conflict between the drug industry's duty to its shareholders (that is, its duty to make money) and its claim to be promoting health and other altruistic ends.

A quick trip to a big drug company's Web site confirms that its stated fundamental responsibility is discovering, developing, and delivering innovative medicines and vaccines that can make a difference in people's lives and create a healthier future. It is, however, according to the financial information also available on the same Web site, a very successful and productive business, with yearly income amounting to several billions of U.S. dollars and a predicted bright financial future.

You don't need a degree in pharmacoeconomics to understand that when multiple drugs, as opposed to single drugs, are recommended in treating health conditions, the drug industry benefits. The elderly, with all their health problems, therefore experience a burden of medication greater than what we would find in a younger person with only a single health problem. Multiple pathology produces multiple prescribing. If the drug industry were ever in a position to promote, produce, encourage, purchase, or otherwise positively influence a drug treatment guideline involving several different medicines, it makes simple sense that the troubled elderly would be affected.

I have heard another cynical argument made, which I mention here because of my attitude toward prevention in the elderly. Imagine that you are an executive in a huge drug corporation who must choose which of two drugs to develop. The budget will be large—$30 million—and the drug not chosen will likely not be developed any time soon. Both drugs have already been studied in a preliminary way.

When you look over the research evidence, you see that the strength of the evidence is about the same for the two drugs.

Both of them have had one or more randomized controlled trials that show that they are better than placebo (better than nothing, that is) for the condition each is designed to treat. But in this imaginary business scenario you were part of the early development, discussions, and studies of these drugs, and you know very well that they are both in fact very nearly useless. Strange to say, useless drugs are produced and sold all the time, as every physician knows. Usually they enjoy a brief heyday of popularity, then fizzle out and get pulled from drug formularies, and in ten years nobody remembers they ever existed.

Two useless drugs, you say to yourself, with just enough evidence to convince academics, government agencies, and payers to take a second look at them. Again, every doctor understands that "false positive" randomized controlled trials exist. I've already suggested several ways that a trial can be unreliable and misleading and still be positive. Nobody in your drug company, least of all you, misrepresented anything with respect to these trials. You have evidence for effectiveness, but you either know or strongly suspect that both drugs are no better than sugar lumps at what they are supposed to do.

Now here's the kicker: drug number one is supposed to control a symptom. This means it is intended to make somebody feeling sick feel better. Let's imagine for the purposes of this scenario that drug number one treats vertigo (dizziness). Drug number two is preventive. It keeps some bad event in the future from happening. Remember, neither of them, really, is effective at all.

Which drug do you choose to spend the $30 million developing? Before continuing, please understand that I'm only imagining what a poisonously cynical critic of the drug industry might try to tell you. No disaffected drug company executive ever anonymously told me about anything of the kind.

Of course you choose drug number two, the preventive drug. Vertigo sufferers would take drug number one for about three days and then throw the rest of the prescription in the garbage, for the good and sufficient reason that the drug doesn't do what it's supposed to and now they know it. But nobody who takes drug number two, the preventive one, ever has any idea that it doesn't work. They keep taking it, and they don't feel any different. Not only is the positive clinical trial that somehow exists all your good well-informed family physician needs to include it in her best-practice care—there is absolutely nothing to oppose it. The drug's alleged benefit may never be falsified. Drug sales will improve, really take off when the drug is included in clinical guidelines for prevention of whatever it "prevents," and fly high indefinitely. At least until the patents on the drug run out.

This is one of the arguments against the drug industry. But if there were any substance to this kind of argument, it would be the frail elderly, who couldn't even benefit from prevention—even if it were actually effective for younger people—who would get disproportionately loaded up with guidelines-mandated pills, and pills, and more pills. There is nothing wrong with prevention in general; some prevention is legitimate—the kind of prevention I would practice myself, for myself. If you're worried about prevention in somebody who isn't a fragile elderly person, sit your doctor down and make sure you understand the situation.

Ethics guidelines for research discourage studies in which one group of subjects receives placebo if there already exists an accepted best-practice treatment for the condition being studied. In plainer language, once a preventive treatment is accepted based on studies that have already been done, you may not be allowed to do a study comparing some preventive treatment to no treatment. It would be considered too dangerous to the people who receive no treatment.

The result of that prohibition on testing "proven" treatments against placebo, again dealt with briefly in Chapter 2, is that it is possible that a worthless preventive treatment not only becomes best practice but gets *locked in* as best practice because once there is a certain amount of evidence for its effectiveness, it can't ethically be studied anymore, and there is no other way of recognizing it is ineffective.

For the reasons I have suggested, and a few other very good ones as well, the drug industry's influence on the medical system can be a very troubling issue, and for some people quite an emotional one. You might be tempted to become suspicious of industry and its motives, and that could spread to (or have already grown out of) a general suspicion of the profit motive. It is a kind of article of faith on the left that business, based on greed and caring nothing for civil rights, human dignity, and stewardship of the environment, will pursue its ends until the whole world is consumed and destroyed. These are concerns that a lot of reasonable people consider real, though not necessarily in their most radical form.

But as a society we have chosen, so far, a free-enterprise way of producing drugs and devices to treat disease. It's there, big as life and playing its role, like it or not. Drug industry is business, but it does over half the health research in Western countries, it produces virtually all the medicines, and it pays for an awful lot of legitimate health education and other health benefits. What would be the alternative? Drug industry run by government? In countries like Canada, where health care is mostly funded by government, there are other problems. And even in such countries, a private-enterprise drug industry continues to supply

medicine, providing the benefits of each corporation's necessity
to compete, while facing government regulation and the rigors
of the marketplace.

If we don't like the way the pharmaceutical industry does
its business, changing it would be a bit like trying to force a big,
wild, carnivorous cat to thrive on a diet of grass and carrots and
then punishing him when he sneaks off and kills a couple of an-
telopes. This problem is not going to go away without a radical
change to the nature of the beast. And any change that makes it
less effective at what it does might make things even worse. This
is a pragmatic point of view. What we have is a long way from
perfect, but it may be the best it can be. I believe in full information advising our opinions. Be careful out there!

Usually second on the list of bad guys when people get together to talk about what's wrong with health care are doctors.
What follows are the usual arguments, not necessarily beliefs I
hold myself. We doctors are not really so bad!

Two classes of doctors come in for a disproportionate dose of
blame: first, the academic leaders, and second, the rank-and-file
generalists out in the trenches. People like me.

Medicine is similar to a lot of other human activities: it's hier-
archical. The general level of academic ability among doctors is
high, guaranteed by extreme competition just to get into medical
school. And so the people at the top of the academic hierarchy in
medicine tend to be pretty remarkable characters. With some exceptions, the majority of these superstars that I have met have a
good practical understanding of where they stand in the pecking
order and a corresponding opinion of themselves.

The most powerful and recognized academic leaders in
any discipline lead and set the standards in teaching, research,
and education administration. They also sit on or chair the

committees and other bodies that review research and set guidelines for clinical practice. These guidelines are very, and increasingly, influential in clinical practice, and so the academic leaders have great influence on the way the rest of us practice.

How does one get to be one of the academic leaders? Presuming industriousness, academic brilliance, political astuteness, and singlemindedness, the answer is really *publication*. I have only a very distant understanding of goings-on in this area, but having sat on a couple of academic search committees, I can say that credibility depends on publishing scholarly articles and in particular on publishing original research.

Publishing in this context doesn't mean getting your name in the morning paper or even writing a book like this one. There are lots of medical and health academic journals, and it is publication in these recognized periodicals that counts. There also exists a hierarchy among the journals. The *New England Journal of Medicine* and the *Journal of the American Medical Association*, for example, are considered prestigious. A paper published in one of these counts for a great deal when an author is being evaluated for a new job or advancement in her department.

Years ago, working with some good friends (some of whom have gone on to the world of academic stardom), I published a research article on the effect of anabolic steroids on healing hip fractures in older people. Our study showed no difference between those who got the steroid and those who got placebo. When we went shopping our research manuscript around to find a publishing journal, a couple of the more important ones turned us down. Now, I'm speculating here, but I don't think this was because we were no-name authors (I certainly was, but I was lucky enough to be working with others who did have names), and I don't think it was because the research was badly done. We had lots of expertise at setting things up in the usual rigorous way. I also think the topic was important. Healing of fractures makes a big difference to outcome in quite a large group of elderly people. And there was lots of biology to suggest that anabolic steroids might make a difference.

No, rejection of our manuscript by the really prestigious publications occurred, I believe, because the study was *negative*—it showed the treatment had no effect. Whether this was true in my case or not, it makes sense that if, because you are recognized as the journal everyone wants to publish in, you have the choice to publish just about any study, and you're going to choose to publish the studies that will have a real impact on clinical practice. The ones that make a difference to treatment and a difference in patients' lives. And in general those are positive studies. Studies that show that something *works*. This is referred to as publication bias, and, like concerns about mixed motives in drug industry, it has been well known and fairly well studied over quite a period of time. But it exists.

Medical research, possibly a bit like the arts, doesn't proceed for free. Although I'm sure many researchers would continue their good work as long as they could even if they weren't paid, recruiting subjects, running research facilities, paying research assistants, and funding all the many consultants you need to do a really big drug trial just costs a lot of money.

I mentioned earlier that the drug industry now funds over half the research done in the Western world. Some estimates put the number as high as 70 percent. Because they stand to benefit directly from positive trials, and because they are big organizations with immense resources, drug companies are a natural to fund drug trials. And the people who do these trials, particularly the people who organize, administer, and lead-author them, tend to be the same prominent academic doctors I've been talking about.

Academic leaders are recognized by publication and then find their way (other things being equal) northward in another hierarchy: medical schools. And so academic excellence tends to concentrate in these cathedrals of health care teaching and research. They are the most difficult schools to enter as a student, and they attract the cream of the crop.

For all these reasons, a concentration of influence rests in the hands of a small number of brilliant, respected, and highly productive people. But for the same reasons, many people unhappy with the current state of health care tend to hold these special doctors responsible.

What's going on when somebody becomes more and more powerful through publishing the results of clinical trials that are positive, rather than negative? What are we supposed to think when the most highly respected professors with the most influence in Western medicine make a significant amount of their income from the drug industry? Journals do publish positive studies preferentially, and nobody can doubt that the drug industry is interested in positive results. The whole thing looks rotten to the core (goes the argument).

Well, it is and it isn't. We can't avoid trusting somebody eventually—or at least, we are willing to delegate certain tasks. We let politicians do the public's business, we let mechanics fix our cars, and we trust our babysitters. We have checks and balances that would prevent somebody really unscrupulous from outrageously abusing that arrangement. Her colleagues would eventually weed her out.

Or would they? Maybe she's only a *little bit* unscrupulous. Possibly the colleagues are not completely vigilant, or are self-interested too. The important idea here boils down to trying to be fair to everybody, I suppose. And with that in mind, I can't escape the worry that these astoundingly successful academic superstar researchers, their work paid for by somebody who benefits from a positive result, and themselves benefiting from a positive result, might face an ethical conflict that even the world's greatest doctors shouldn't have to confront. And the result of that, over time, would be more prevention, more medication, more rigid guidelines, and a more uncompromising, dangerous, and irrelevant style of medical care for the fragile elderly. Goes the argument.

At the other end of the academic hierarchy, way down at the bottom of the totem pole, crouch we primary care doctors. And I can state from long personal experience that some comfort comes from having a view parallel to the horizon and your feet close to the ground. But the cartoon of the ordinary doctor applies only in a very general way. And what I'm going to say about the way the world blames us general practitioners is what the general view is, not what I really believe.

The first time I read Ivan Illich's book *Medical Nemesis,* I realized he was on to something. The quote at the start of this chapter says much of it. I've seen other general practitioners or family doctors do things that went well above and beyond being "an artisan exercising a skill on personally known individuals." People who agonize over unexplained weight loss, suffer when their patients are depressed, get involved in unusual specific treatment strategies, and insist on making sure that specialists know and understand the information they need to help with a difficult case exist among the doctors I work with. They make the rest of us look good. And they make us proud.

But as I have already described, the tendency is away from this kind of personal responsibility and more toward meeting a standard defined by a guideline. Students (held, if possible, in even lower esteem than primary care doctors) were abused by teachers in a different way when I was in medical school. The expectation was that we would assume responsibility, and we were (at least I was) held up to ridicule if we didn't respond to late-night calls immediately, explore every possibility in making a diagnosis, and carefully explain everything to family members. But today's teachers insist instead on uniform application of diagnostic and treatment guidelines above all else.

The difference may not be obvious to a patient. But today the average general practitioner slogging it out in his storefront in the mall or in her tenth-storey office is encouraged to deal with heart failure, for example, according to a very strict set of rules. The rules involve making a diagnosis using technology, looking for beside-the-point risk factors (smoking, high cholesterol, diet, and so on), encouraging "lifestyle" changes, and then, most important, prescribing *all* the preventive medications. Nowhere on the form that doctors are now encouraged to fill out (in my community, to receive a payment bonus for following the guidelines) is there anything about what the patient's priorities are, whether the patient belongs to the population the guidelines were designed for, how the patient feels about the diagnosis, and whether the patient wants to get better.

This isn't all bad, of course. Practicing consistently probably coincides with a measurable benefit to the population of people with an illness. But an important baby goes out with the bathwater of inconsistent practice. Inconsistency in practice partly exists because there really is inconsistency among people. When we treat everyone the same, we endorse the idea that everyone *is* the same.

How much energy do we have? For me, it's eventually limited. After adhering exactly to a consistent set of rules, I may not have enough psychological zip—or time—left at the end of an appointment or a long day to ask a patient how he feels, what he thinks about what I'm telling him, whether anything else is bothering him, or whether he even gives a damn. At the same time I'm encouraged to consider my job well done once that consistent set of rules is followed.

Nevertheless, switching to that guidelines-oriented standard can be a huge relief. Just how comprehensive a saint am I expected to be, grinding away in the trenches of my office in the mall?

And that, finally, is the awful truth about what Ivan Illich is saying. A consistent, cookbook practice is *easier*. The average doctor I see around me in general practice is a tidy, organized, hardworking person much more at home with something that can be defined and limited than with the awful open-endedness of responsibility for what happens to somebody. Who isn't? The criticism that might be directed at us, down on our haunches at the bottom of the totem pole, is that we abandon people in favor of a set of rules. We might reply that we're just following orders, and indeed we are. But that argument is suspect as well.

So we followers among doctors, the people to whom the guidelines are directed, may stand to be accused of complicity with the new consistent health care. Nothing wrong with that, unless the idea I'm selling you in this book holds some water. If it's true that fragile old people are all individuals in many important ways and that their needs are met only through understanding their individuality, then we primary care prescribers, in always carefully following general guidelines, would be as guilty as anyone of preventing them from getting what they need.

As I have said, however, this is a trend, and doctors remain who still remember why they chose to do this job and still suffer in sympathy with unhappy people every day.

Last in the usual lineup when we go looking for who is to blame for the medical system's troubles are administrators. Not just the people themselves, but the corporate structures, public or private, that produce a different set of rules than academic doctors do. These are rules to do with payment. And the criticism they face is predictably of the form, "Who cares what it costs? This is my (leg, life, vision, fertility, sanity) we're talking about here!"

But health care is expensive, and it's getting worse. The cost of everything involved in looking after people seems to increase out of line with inflation or with anything else. Drug costs are ballooning. The increase in hospital costs per day outstrips pretty well every other comparable service business. The equipment, the vehicles, and the people command high—and rising— prices. The population changes, featuring greater numbers of very old people suffering from greater numbers of costly conditions compound this problem. Statistics suggest that the percentage of the gross domestic product devoted to health care is increasing in practically all Western countries. Although these countries differ in how much they spend on health care, all are spending more and more.

So at the same time that medical care is becoming increasingly rigid and prescriptive in its form, there is increasingly an unavoidable concern with cost. And it's not nurses, consumers, doctors, or drug industry sales staff who carry the responsibility for this scary reality. It's administrators.

So who are these administrators? In general they work in government departments or for health care insurers, health maintenance organizations, drug plans, and other payers. And perfectly appropriately, the people in charge of this activity of examining, controlling, rationalizing, and distributing cost are people trained in business. Bean counters.

How are decisions about payment made? Typically, big health care payers will have medical consultants, a job I've also done and still do. They pay people like me to give advice on medical questions. But whether administrators listen to that medical advice or not, decisions about what to pay for and how much to pay fall to them, with their business training.

Those decisions about payment must be justified in some way. Whether we are making decisions about benefits paid for by government or by an insurance company, people receiving those benefits are entitled to consistency and some sort of a rational process. How come Harry got the titanium glasses and I had to make do with plastic? Why did I have to wait for my MRI when the halfback on the other team had his right away? I've got cancer: how long do I have to wait for my operation? Putting ourselves in the place of the person who has to respond to this kind of question, we're going to avoid making discretionary decisions ourselves. We need a set of rules.

As we have seen, sets of rules for medical practice certainly exist, and their effect is to encourage consistency of treatment.

And it happens that the need for consistency in health care administration, to keep it from appearing arbitrary, generally is met by these sets of rules or guidelines. One way to reinforce consistency in care is to teach the rules in professional education. But a separate and very powerful way is to pay only for care that follows those rules. And this is the consequence when the health care administration naturally and unavoidably embraces cookbook treatment. We get only guideline care because that's the kind that's paid for.

The drug industry has, many people would allege, an influence on clinical guidelines. No academic committee can recommend a treatment that industry doesn't produce. The drugs that are developed are the drugs that are projected to be profitable for the producer. Ideally, we might imagine, these would be the drugs for which there is a need, and everything is fine. Sick people out there have unmet needs, industry produces effective treatment, drugs sell like hotcakes, everybody's happy.

But industry seeks and pays for information about which drugs, at what price, and with which kinds of clinical trial findings, payers will fund. This is part of reasonable business strategy. To some extent, then, the drugs that get produced are the drugs that industry believes will be accepted for payment. But remember, clinical guidelines can only include drugs that exist— that is, drugs that industry is producing. And the guidelines in turn define what insurers will pay for.

If we use our skeptical imagination a little, we might find support for a paranoid conspiracy theory. Research academics need to do studies and so go looking for funding, industry provides it as long as they study the drugs industry intends to produce, and industry listens carefully to what the public and private drug plans will cover. But at the bottom of this merry-go-round is a characteristic that meets the need of nearly everyone on board: consistency.

Give us rules to base our payment on. Make the rules consistent. Let's not have exceptions that lead to complaints of favoritism, arbitrary decision making, and unreasonableness. Make sure our lawyers can convince a judge that we apply the same set of rules for payment to everybody. Now *there's* a set of demands both compelling and relatively easy to follow. Compelling because the demand is coming from the person with the money. The *consumer*, in aggregate. Easy to follow because the whole evidence-based movement with its guidelines is already oriented that way. Everything feeds on consistency. Goes the argument.

Imagine the problems people with business training trying to run a consistent payment program would have if somebody insisted that they fund caring, kindness, common sense, and other forms of responsible hand-holding by health professionals. (Institutional payers rarely see the actual care they're paying for.) Imagine if they had to listen to the quirky requests and demands of oddball people who didn't conform to any kind of rule that would allow them to make a reasonable decision whether to pay or not. What would happen if they had to choose, with nothing else but a piece of paper to go by, between paying a massage therapist who is honestly making a person in pain feel better and another one who is pretty much operating a brothel? Unless they had rules of evidence about massage they'd have no way of telling the difference. I don't think even the most angry critic of health care administration could suggest putting administrators in that kind of position.

The point is that health care administration's need for consistency has imparted a little extra spin, or a lot of spin, to the self-reinforcing cycle of cookbook care. Administrators wouldn't be able to function if they couldn't use a "reliable" set of rules. That is, if they had to identify care that really works for each client.

So we see that influences in medical care exist to promote the cookbook approach to treatment. And I think it is our tendency, whether we are caregivers, doctors, nurses, or anybody else involved with a fragile old person, to jump to some easy conclusions about why the medical system isn't reaching those people the way it should. The drug industry, various kinds of doctors, and administrators who pay the bills all play a role in making things more difficult.

It really would be wonderful to righteously grip one or more of these obvious villains by the lapels and pull him up out of his dirty hiding place into the light for us all to recognize, blame, and punish. Filthy drug industry, ignoring the needs of pathetic old people in its greed. Megalomaniac or moronically consistent doctors playing along with industry and blindly following a set of rules. Administrators who are even further from considering individual patients' needs, completely preoccupied with balancing a budget and staying out of trouble. I'd love to do that, but I just can't. I have worked with people from all of these groups, and all I can say is that most of them are doing the best they can, most with a reasonable and generally acceptable amount of self-interest, and circumstances have simply drifted into the ugly and dangerous mess I'm worried about.

But wait a minute. When we think about it, isn't there one other group of people who benefit from a straightforward, simple, easy-to-follow approach to looking after difficult and complicated health care problems? To quote Pogo: "We have met the enemy, and he is us." Ordinary people getting old, or with relatives getting old. Bless our hearts.

Truly, it is so much easier to press a button or go for a ready-made solution when faced with hard choices, awkward people, old conflicts, and the extent of our own responsibility. Easier than changing our worldview or even having a difficult conversation with Mum or Dad, especially if they're not so good at hearing or understanding what we're talking about. Then it's more like a difficult conversation with *ourselves,* which can be the worst kind. But just possibly it is to ourselves that we have to look if we're serious about keeping old folks out of trouble.

A doctor friend in an unaccustomed philosophical mood said to me recently, "We get the kind of health care we deserve." Deserve? The last two chapters of this book are about deciding what that health care could look like and mulling over whether we're ready to think about the care of old people in a completely different way.

# 9 Nobody Asked Us
## What Fragile Old People Want and Need

ANN DAVENPORT

Dr. Davenport, who holds a PhD in American fiction, always refuses to take any medication. She is eighty-two and very frail, barely able to get to the bathroom with her walker. When I did get her to agree to a blood test, her thyroid function was definitely low, and, as I told her many times, this could be improved by taking a thyroid hormone replacement pill. But she wasn't interested. I suggested her energy level might be better with treatment, but she preferred to chat about Nathaniel Hawthorne. Many times, in my hurry to get through the afternoon, I left her tiny apartment feeling guilty because I had cut short a fascinating conversation we were both enjoying. Business is business.

But one time, she kept me talking for over an hour when we got on the subject of what she wanted out of life. I was astounded that though this lady was not depressed (she was the farthest thing from depressed), she would quite happily have chosen to have her life end quietly that very night. What is it about the future causing her to prefer not to experience it? I wondered. So I asked her.

"My daughter is doing too much for me already. She does all my shopping, takes care of the banking, and checks on me every day. She works full time. Sometimes she has to clean up when I don't make it to the bathroom, and I see the look on her face. The most important thing to me is, I don't want to die with somebody I love hating what they have to do for me. I've had a great life. Now it's over."

### EMIL SCHOENFELD

A few weeks after my fascinating visit with Dr. Davenport I visited ninety-eight-year-old Mr. Schoenfeld in his assisted-living apartment. I had been preoccupied with the idea that an apparently mentally healthy old person might prefer not to go on living, and I had asked several patients about that. I got some surprising answers. On this visit I had a medical student with me and had explained to her my finding about old people's wishes for the future. Thinking to show her a real-life example, I asked Mr. Schoenfeld whether he would take an opportunity not to wake up in the morning, if he had one.

"No way!" he said, charmingly using contemporary slang with his strong Austrian accent. A bit taken aback, I asked why not. "I might miss something," was the reply.

### ELZBIETA KALINSKA

Mrs. Kalinska redefines histrionic. Whenever anything is wrong—and whenever nothing is wrong—she shouts and gesticulates about the horror of her life. Her voice is scratchy and pathetic, her facial expression one of unimaginable suffering. The complaint usually starts with something that sounds legitimately health related: pain, change in the bowels, inability to get to sleep. But within a sentence or two it has moved over into what really counts: Mrs. Kalinska has been betrayed by her family, treated like a concentration camp prisoner in the hospital, and insulted by worthless, lazy home support workers. The world is garbage; imagine the impropriety of her having to live in it!

At one point she complained of a painful rash, which when I visited her I confirmed was shingles. On the next visit she still had it, and it was still painful (as anybody who's ever had shingles knows). She was taking a lot more than her usual three or four Tylenol No. 3s per day. But something was subtly less hysterical: she asked me if it would be okay to show me her painted handkerchiefs. Normally I'd beg off because of not enough time, but that day I didn't have the heart. What beautiful linen handkerchiefs, perfectly folded, with charming, precise floral work in the center and around the edge. There was something really arresting about the wild symmetrical colors of each of them as she threw them on the couch.

I was surprised at my disappointment that she didn't offer me one. There was a soft look in her eyes I'd never seen before as she told me how much she loves it when she and her friend, who visits her several times a week, make and admire these hankies. This very difficult lady has something many of my other patients need: a valued relationship and a way to maintain self-respect. Somebody who cares and something to live for.

IT CAN BE difficult to put yourself in someone else's shoes. We are all inclined to assume that others see the world through the same eyes we do. What do old people want at the end of their lives? A very similar situation to the one I described at the beginning of Chapter 1 exists here, I think. Yes, there are general answers to this question, but we have to recognize that the people we are talking about are all so different from one another that the specifics are going to be quirky and unpredictable. By now, this is not unexpected.

Scientific health care delivers consistent care and prevention of, and rescue from, death—what most younger people are looking for. These things are not what fragile old people want at all.

The needs and desires of fragile old people often involve what will happen to them while they are dying. "End-of-life" is one name we give to the topic of death and dying in health care. We are interested in the wants and needs of a group of people who are near the end of life. Dying is a real and important matter for just about all very elderly people. And what they want is of great interest to everybody. Does the information available about this subject apply in my practice?

Yes and no. Some of the well-known descriptions of the dying process only make sense in certain situations. Elisabeth Kübler-Ross's famous model, involving stages of thinking about dying that culminate in acceptance, fits best when people know they are going to die, know approximately when it's going to happen, and stay reasonably mentally alert. A cancer death in an otherwise healthy person, for example.

Although death is often looked at as a routine matter in hospitals, it has never become routine for me, even though I've cared for hundreds of people at the time of their deaths. And my patients don't tend to fit models of death and dying.

Palliative care is now a well-established part of health care. According to its philosophy, death and dying are taken to be natural, very real, of course inevitable, and coming up in a clearly defined period of time. The difference between the palliative population and the people in my practice has to do with *when* people are expected to die. Palliative patients are traditionally expected to die in under six months. With my patients, we usually don't really know. They are near the end of their life, but how near?

There's another, more important difference than timing between palliative care patients and the people I see. One of the goals of palliative care is to provide patients with a comfortable, dignified death. And this goal is very often met for palliative patients. Pain is controlled, psychological comfort is provided, and there is a sense of understanding and completion when someone dies. There is, if one can put it this way, a certain *orderliness* to good palliative care. The patients tend in a general way to experience the Kübler-Ross changes of preparing for death, and then the interventions of palliative care are effective enough that they die comfortably and with dignity.

I should parenthetically clarify the idea of "death with dignity." The phrase has come to be associated with legislation permitting euthanasia. I'm not talking about that fascinating and terribly controversial subject here but about the circumstances surrounding natural death in fragile elderly people.

Most of the people I have cared for who die wouldn't be classified as palliative care patients at all. The majority of the deaths I'm aware of have been either slow, or fairly quick as a result of a crisis. Death in my practice seems to happen as part of the gradual-deterioration-with-crises picture I've already tried to describe. Once in a while a frail elderly person just dwindles away. Other times some sort of a crisis occurs, and death happens, or is allowed to happen, in that setting. You may recall Mrs.

Chau—the difficult and unwell lady who fairly suddenly got sick and needed us to decide whether she should go to the hospital. That kind of crisis and that kind of outcome are common.

A doctor I know who practices in my community, David Kuhl, has written a wonderful book, *What Dying People Want*. This well-researched book is based on an original study of the needs and desires among palliative patients. What emerges is that people near the end of life are looking for meaning and spiritual reassurance. Because death for a nonpalliative elderly person may take a long time, and he may have bed sores, problems with the bowels and urine, and sometimes a need for many months of heavy care in bed, it can be even more difficult to offer that kind of help than it is with the true palliative patient. There's no question in my mind that dying people want meaning and spirituality. But how to achieve it under the circumstances of my patients?

A patient of mine who died recently was a retired engineer who spent a total of four years in an extended care unit. He entered this facility after he suffered a stroke that caused him to lose his mobility and most of his ability to communicate in words. His family was kind and patient to the end, but I knew how hard it was for his wife to come to the nursing home month after month, seeing her husband suffer, never really sure if he even recognized who she was. This man had a lot of pain (he had a condition called polymyalgia rheumatica, which he developed before he had his stroke) and had to take a corticosteroid, which made in his skin very fragile, along with morphine. I tried everything I could think of to control the pain without side effects. Nurses at the facility were wonderful about his wounds. But all his care was complicated by "double incontinence" (no control of the bowels or the urine), which again was very stubborn and resisted our best evaluation and treatment efforts. He died of a pneumonia, which, following some terrible soul-searching by his wife, was not treated.

People in my practice usually die either slowly over a long time, like this patient, or as part of a crisis. But beyond that I see all sorts of circumstances. Over half my patients who die, die in "delirium." That is, they are unaware or only partly aware of what's happening at the time of their death. This is consistent with studies on the subject. Many patients, especially people who have been demented or very immobile for a long time, are just found dead in the morning.

The reason dignity while dying may be very hard to accomplish when one of my patients dies is familiar: unpredictability. There isn't time to organize the wonderful interventions of palliative care in a crisis situation. And psychological and physical comfort can be hard to sustain where someone dies over quite a long time, during which the kind of problems my retired engineer patient experienced can challenge the most dedicated caregivers.

I'll close this discussion of end of life by describing one of my patients (who, as it happens, is still alive). Emily Martin, who has Parkinson's disease, is typically atypical. This incredibly sad woman is only in her late forties, but her disease is so severe that she is terribly disabled. She has had every kind of medical care available—seen all the medical experts and undergone the latest and best of available surgical treatments, too (she was one of the first people to have a brain stimulator implanted to treat her Parkinson's disease).

Emily's husband, Dan, is an extremely energetic man who loves his wife dearly. For many years he has been her main caregiver. At one point, frustrated with the inability of local experts to help his wife, he took her to a special clinic he found on the Internet, where she had further surgery. The result was some improvement in her awful symptoms but also complete loss of her ability to speak.

Emily sits in a chair all day, fed by a home support helper, and suffers from severe stiffness and spasms of her muscles. This comes partly from the Parkinson's disease and partly from the medications she must take. The expression on her face and the sometimes difficult-to-decipher signals she provides are the only indication we have of how she is doing. She is very thin; her face seems to be all eyes, with her mouth pulled into a grimace. Many times I have visited her and been aware of her intelligent, frightened gaze fixed on me. We in my business try to be objective, but I always find Emily's mute, remote hopefulness incredibly disturbing.

A couple of years ago a kind of crisis occurred where Emily seemed to be in much worse pain than usual nearly all the time, was having trouble swallowing, and was quickly losing weight. It looked for a while as if she might die from malnutrition and dehydration and also as if she was going to die in pain.

I had tried every possible pain treatment I could think of, none of which seemed to help. I called one of my palliative care colleagues, a wonderful creative doctor who visited my patient and then suggested treatment. Tiny doses of hydromorphone, an opioid (narcotic) medicine, were his suggestion (I had tried a more conventional dose, which she couldn't tolerate). Emily did seem to have some relief with these. Unfortunately, husband Dan was still concerned about side effects of drowsiness, and so eventually he had to stop giving her the drug. I don't know how Emily survived this difficult time. Somehow her swallowing improved, and the awful expressions of pain seemed to get a little better as well. But at times her life has seemed like one crisis after another.

How long will Emily live? And what will her death be like? *And what does she want?* As I've said, it's very hard to know. But keeping her comfortable, maintaining communication, and somehow trying to prevent her from losing herself in terrible desperation are difficult problems that never go away. And we have to just presume that these would be her priorities.

Where preparing for death is concerned, what people want sometimes depends on how much they know. Are fragile old people aware of what is likely to happen to them in advance? I think this is also variable. Scholarly articles argue both sides of the question, but the picture I see among my patients predictably defies generalization. What does a very demented person know or think about the future? Will elderly people necessarily tell us what's on their minds, where dying is concerned? This characteristic of being near the end of life is not something anyone can change. And the question of how aware somebody is of being near the end of life will always have an individual answer. Some people understand they are going to die soon. Some people manage by maintaining ambivalence, or even denial, which might not be such a bad strategy. But all cope in the way their life experience and personality, the situation they're in, and the people around them allow.

Here's what my experience tells me, allowing for how different everyone is, about what old people think and know about death. First, yes, most who are aware of their circumstances do know that they are old and that, being old, they are likely to die sooner rather than later. Second, they tend to have reached some sort of comfort with that fact.

But on this terribly serious topic, I find strange and even humorous situations that defy long-faced scholarly generalities. I want to tell you a quick story about my own father. My dad was not at all a frail elderly person. About ten days before he died at the age of seventy-five, he was driving around town, working on a real estate project, and playing golf. One night while he was visiting a nearby city with my stepmother, he called my brother and me very late at night complaining of chest pain. It was, unhappily, a serious heart attack, and he had more heart trouble on his second day in the hospital. The last night, with all of the family there, poor Dad had five or six cardiac arrests. Each time, the intensive care unit nurses called the intern, and I had the quite horrifying experience of watching this very young doctor manage the resuscitation and then the even worse one of helping decide whether to try to resuscitate my dear old dad the next time.

After the last resuscitation my brother and I were holding our dad's hands and talking to him. He had had some morphine; he was in and out of consciousness. Suddenly, he looked at us both and said, "God damn it: you have to die five times!"

This was both perfectly typical of our dad's dry sense of humor and a very clear advance directive. With the next cardiac arrest, about twenty minutes later, he got a little bit of intravenous morphine and no resuscitation attempt. He finally died peacefully.

I remember another strange death decision. Victor Morales, age ninety-nine, was meticulously looked after at home by his daughter, Maria. She lived upstairs; he was in the basement. Mr. Morales was very frail and needed help to be transferred from bed to the toilet or to a chair. Maria had a no-nonsense home support worker every day to assist with this and with feeding her father. I said Maria took meticulous care, but sometimes I wondered how realistic she was. Whenever Mr. Morales sneezed (I mean this almost literally), I would get a phone call. Since I had taken over his care, however, Maria had stopped calling an ambulance and rushing him to the hospital on each of these occasions. Calling me instead looked like progress.

I prescribed antibiotics regularly for Mr. Morales's frequent chest infections, even though most of them were caused by his choking on a little bit of liquid if he wasn't very carefully fed. He had had several strokes. Maria always insisted that her dad wanted to survive no matter what. Although he couldn't speak, when I asked him about this, he vigorously nodded his head. I assumed there was some religious consideration involved, and of course I went along with his stated wishes.

Unfortunately, I was out of town and so missed Victor Morales's hundredth birthday party, to which I was invited. I heard the food was incredible. Three weeks later Mr. Morales suddenly got short of breath and started coughing, and Maria called me. I offered to visit him and to prescribe the usual antibiotics, but she surprised me by saying, "No, I think we'll just keep him comfortable."

Victor Morales just wanted to be a hundred years old, and he made it.

On the subject of dying, I have no choice but to offer up a non-answer to the question of what old people want: all sorts of different things. But consistently, they want us to *listen*. And I think it's fair to say nearly all of them don't want to be left alone.

When we try to understand the answer to the general question of what old people want, some useful information comes from looking at preferences that elderly, fragile elderly, and dying people state formally. These are usually referred to as "advance directives" or "living wills." The idea here is that while we are still mentally capable, we get to tell other people what we would like done in various possible situations if we are ever not able to make or communicate decisions ourselves.

Many places have laws defining what is a legitimate advance directive and what isn't. Whether they are written down or reliably communicated in words to someone, advance wishes tend to be respected by the courts. But it's very rare for this kind of thing to be tested in court. Much more commonly a form has been filled out, at home or in a nursing home, which nurses, ambulance drivers, doctors, and others get a chance to look at so that they can follow the directions in a crisis. Whether to resuscitate in the event of a cardiac arrest, transfer to hospital, put the person on a respirator, or provide artificial feeding, as well as how to deal with a range of other predictable situations, may be included. Most of my patients have their advance directive forms stuck on the front of their fridge.

Several living will packages, as I think of them, exist in books, online, for free, and for sale. I find they tend to include too much detail. Most elderly people and their families have trouble picturing and describing what kind of loss of function would be unacceptable to them and don't really understand the difference between, say, tube feeding and supplemental feeding. These things can be explained, of course, but another problem with detailed advance directives is that they really never foresee exact events or the flavor of any crisis. What's happened in the last several days, how does everybody in the family feel, who's in town, exactly what resources are available, how crowded is the emergency room at the moment, is it just before or just after Christmas, and so on.

To help people through a crisis, I need to know in general whether a person favors comfort or prolonging life (if we must choose between the two) and who the trusted substitute decision maker would be if the person were not able to decide for himself. I can't remember a situation requiring a difficult decision that wasn't covered by the answers to those two questions.

I have to just say a quick word about cardiac arrest resuscitation. Most readers will be familiar with this procedure through the media: when someone collapses, has no pulse, and is not breathing, another person pushes on the victim's chest and puffs air into her mouth to artificially support breathing and circulation. Eventually an attempt is made to shock the heart back into functioning rhythm, and drugs are given.

For fragile old people, studies show universally bad outcomes even in the best of circumstances. A small number of people survive cardiac arrest, but most of them suffer brain damage or damage to other vital organs.

For that reason I advise my patients and their families not to request cardiac arrest resuscitation in their advance directives. Perhaps my views are colored a little by my own father's experience. It just doesn't seem worthwhile for people's last experience on earth to include someone crunching away on their chest and (as soon as the ambulance arrives) getting the front of their body sizzled with four hundred watt-seconds of direct current. Is this kind of abuse worth it to obtain brain-damaged survival for a small number of folks? Not for me, thanks. But for people who understand what's going on and do want resuscitation, I do my very best to see that they get it.

At any rate, when we study advance directives, what do we find out about preferences? Many years ago I asked the "comfort versus prolonging life" question to about twenty elderly people in nursing homes. I published the result: all but one (95 percent) favored comfort over prolonging life.

And this finding is consistent with other studies. People making these decisions in advance generally want pain controlled and don't want to be kept alive artificially. *But there are exceptions.* In the relevant literature there is a consensus that prevention of and rescue from death are far down the list of preferences and desires among people who understand that for them, time may be short. So what is it they do want?

Another anecdote may help us. Maggie Dunlop was the sister of one of my former schoolteachers. She had come from Australia to be with what was left of her family and apparently had a more than adequate family fortune to set her up in a nice big condominium apartment with round-the-clock caregivers. When I first met her, she was charming and polite and told me everything was just fine. But over the next few weeks it became obvious that she suffered from terrible, chronic pain. The source of this pain was obscure. My evaluation suggested it was coming from her brain, the result of a stroke she had had. Written consultations from specialists in Australia, which arrived eventually and were very thorough, didn't really clarify things much.

Maggie had lots of trouble getting around. Her home support worker helped her, but it was also painful for her to walk. Being in pain all the time was not good for her mood. She didn't enjoy anything very much, and she admitted she felt blue and depressed nearly all the time.

She was taking several drugs for pain and depression when I started seeing her, but they weren't working. To make a long and difficult story short, after I made sure that there weren't any causes of the pain I could fix, I tried every pain medication in the book, carefully, one at a time and in combination, and up to absolutely maximum doses, but nothing seemed to work. Week after week my promises that we would find something effective sounded less and less convincing. Several times Maggie told me she would rather be dead than suffer with the pain she was experiencing.

When she developed a bad chest infection, she was hospitalized and seen by a hospital pain specialist. She was in the hospital for a couple of months, and when she finally came out, the pain was about the same and her mobility was quite a bit worse. I had mixed feelings about the hospital pain experts' failure: I regretted that they couldn't help her, but at least I hadn't missed anything.

I wish there were a happy ending to Maggie's story. The last time I saw her, the family was about to move her to a nursing home outside the city, and I transferred her records to a different doctor. I hope he had better success helping her, but I'm afraid I doubt it.

The tone of Maggie Dunlop's situation is much different from that of Dr. Davenport's, but the pattern is similar: a situation for each of them worse than death, in its way. These are two people who don't have what they want and need. Dr. Davenport needs to not be a burden on her daughter, whom she loves, and Mrs. Dunlop needs to not suffer with an intolerable symptom nobody can fix. Neither of them is the least bit interested in preventing a heart attack or taking their multiple vitamins to maintain their bone density. Neither would go anywhere near a hospital if they could help it. They have much more important priorities on their mind.

Another need, and also a very frequently expressed desire among fragile elderly people that I see at home, is to be treated as a self. As a person. It seems incredible even to have to say this, but it's equally incredible how often, in my experience, the humanity of someone who can't effectively demand respect from others is violated or just plain ignored.

This is one of the reasons it is important for fragile old people not to go to the hospital. Elizabeth O'Malley, for example, whose story appeared at the start of Chapter 2, didn't need to be in the hospital and had some ugly and scary medical trouble because of being there, for technical reasons to do with her heart. But more than that, she was disturbed by *the way she felt she was treated.*

Her description of her time in the hospital was that she hated every minute of it. She told me that people (doctors, nurses, laboratory personnel, *everybody*) treated her "as if I wasn't there." I tried to get her to discuss this (and to tell me who the people were), but she didn't really want to talk about it and just insisted that she would never go back there again.

I don't know quite what has happened lately to morale in hospitals in North America and, I'm sure, elsewhere in the world. Although lots of exceptions exist, morale is generally low. The problem is not so much that people working in hospitals don't like their jobs, are underpaid, or are somehow subject to mood disorders but rather that these capable, trained people have to do things they know are futile and may in fact be making somebody's life worse. The picture of Mrs. O'Malley in a cardiac care unit is for me an emblem of the poor fit between people and care that is the subject of this book. And I feel as much sympathy and sadness for the people who work in hospitals as for the elderly patients who get stuck there. I imagine many of them saying to themselves, "It wasn't supposed to be like this!" This reminds me of how I felt about practicing medicine when I was working in a city office: I signed up to *help* people. How come I'm spending my time doing *this*?

This is not to diminish the commitment, effort (sometimes lifelong), and caring that many wonderful hospital professionals give, often thanklessly and anonymously. The same thing applies to some family doctors I know who actually love city office practice. When I started out in family practice, I was teamed with a much older man, about the age I am now, who was a wonderful GP. Several times when I felt discouraged, I would sit and talk to him about next to nothing for ten minutes and just feel better. He was the kind of doctor people went to see just for that reason; his *medical* work didn't matter much by comparison.

Working at systematically applying remedies that we know perfectly well the people we care for don't want, need, or benefit from isn't good for job satisfaction. Whatever profession we're in, mindlessly applying guidelines and clinical pathways to people whose priorities are in a completely different universe can make agents of grief out of the very best of us, or at least bore us to tears. At the same time, you can't have an effective hospital without guidelines and clinical pathways, and you can't do effective preventive general practice without them either.

But back to the psychological side of Elizabeth O'Malley's experience of the hospital. Fortunately she got out and stayed out. Many other old people aren't as lucky. Many die in the hospital, and of course the morale-destroying futility of caring for someone who is in the hospital for reasons that don't make any sense is compounded as it becomes clear that they're not going to get out. Treated like she "wasn't there"—what a way to die!

The elderly people in my practice aren't telling me about what they need but about a lot of things they *don't* need: they very badly want and need to *not* be a burden on loved ones, to *not* face intolerable symptoms, and to *not* be treated as if they aren't a person, a self.

The fragile elderly are all different from one another, and they also feel differently about relationships with other people. I've seen quiet old people who are perfectly happy being left alone get driven to distraction by well-meaning but insensitive helpers who haul them off to adult day centers so that they won't be lonely. But others really are isolated and frightened, frozen behind shutters of pride and fear of being a burden. I always struggle with the constraints of my work. Getting around to see everybody, calling the pharmacy, and answering the pager make it hard for me to meet that kind of social need myself. There are times when I think I should be spending an hour or two having tea with somebody instead of dealing with their diabetes, bowel movements, breathlessness, and medication and then getting out the door so that I can fit another six people into the afternoon.

What can we do about an old person who is lonely and depressed, feels isolated, and doesn't have any friends? Go and visit them, of course. But predictably, there are problems with this. How do we know the person *wants* to be visited? What kind of visitor would help, and is that particular kind of visitor available? And—to me most annoying and difficult of all—we run into the perception that because it is pretty well impossible to do a scientific study of the benefit of visiting, you can't prove its value. Therefore it isn't in the health care mainstream, nobody really takes it seriously, and there is no point in spending any money on it. Worse, well-motivated academic people try to be scientific anyway and produce and publish some of the most inconclusive contradictory nonsense imaginable, which just reinforces cynicism about trying to help isolated people.

This is another example of how in modern health care we tend to moronically turn every question into a scientific one when the answer may be staring us in the face and at the same time may be inaccessible to the methods of science. Yes, loneliness is a complicated, difficult problem. And no, like just about everything else to do with this disorderly group of elderly people, you can't do a watertight scientific study of it. But the problem, if anybody can do anything about it at all, is so plainly and obviously amenable to common sense and just a little human sensitivity that trying to be scientific about it properly looks ridiculous.

Frank Hamaguchi was a retired logger who lived in a tiny bachelor apartment on the sixteenth floor of a subsidized seniors' highrise. He was eighty-four but only just lately had started to get a little forgetful and begun to fall. He'd had four falls, two of them bad enough that he was picked up off the street and taken to the hospital. No serious injuries, except to his pride. His parents emigrated from Japan many years ago, and he was raised in the Pacific Northwest. Frank came across as the gruff, strong, and silent type, very much the bush bachelor in town. But he loved classical music and had strong and (to me) reasonable ideas about government and human nature. A complicated guy wrapped in a rigid, traditional shell.

As I got to know him, tried to help with his urinary incontinence (the apartment stank, unfortunately), and worked on fixable causes of his falling, it gradually dawned on me that Frank missed the fellowship that existed in the logging camps. "None of the goddamn people in this place will talk to you," he told me.

I contacted a local volunteer organization, and a very nice older-middle-aged lady phoned Frank and came to visit him. The next time I saw him, he was really angry at me. "Was it you that sent that syrupy bitch over here?" Things had not gone well.

The truth, as everybody appreciates, is that helping someone without providing something substantive, like flat tire repair or pills for their stomachache, is extremely difficult to do. Lonely, socially isolated people don't have old friends, so the person cold-calling and walking in the door is a stranger. The implied contract is almost impossible for either of the two people to deal with: "You poor lonely old person. I'm here to be nice to you because I'm nice. Presumably something is wrong with you, which we hope an hour of being exposed to *me* can fix. Let's be friends," would be how the lonely old person perceives it. Anyone who has ever tried to do this recognizes the problem. It's one thing to help someone by offering some specific service but an entirely different proposition to try to help by offering *yourself*.

A wonderful long-term-care case manager suggested Frank attend a card group for older, retired working men. It turned out to be a perfect fit, and I think he's still attending it. He was falling, by the way, because of low blood pressure, which I was able to fix.

Hannah Eichel is an old woman (ninety-one), whom a home care nurse originally called me to see because Hannah was "difficult." She refuses treatment, she refuses diagnosis, she refuses to quit smoking, she refuses to eat properly, and she's stuck in bed because her arms and legs are weak for reasons that nobody can figure out. Her apartment is kept reasonably clean by daily home support workers, who also prepare food. A truce had been reached: Hannah wanted strictly pizza and ice cream, and this was what she got, since she went on a hunger semistrike and nearly died last year.

Very crotchety and eccentric, Hannah always engages me with an ironic barroom-babe act like some character out of Bertolt Brecht. "So are we going to Las Vegas this weekend, honey?" She watches a black-and-white television and reads a kind of romance fiction that I didn't think existed anymore. Her cigarette smoking worries everyone. She has no family, no friends, and no visitors except professionals and the home support worker. When I tried to organize volunteers to chat with her (and when I tried to mobilize her and figure out why she was immobile) she always said, "Baby, *I just want to be left alone!*" And she does. Alone in the world and isolated, but happy.

Imagine trying to do a scientific study of the effect or effectiveness of visits, adult day centers, socialization groups, outings, and other social interventions on socially isolated old people like Frank and Hannah. What do you "measure"? A depression scale? Score on a questionnaire about how things are going? Admission to hospital? How many times someone smiles or cries in a one-hour interview? And what, really, is the "intervention"? A dear, well-meaning older member of the opposite sex with very limited social skills comes to call, for example?

Searching the scholarly literature using key words like "aged," "elderly," "the frail," "home visit," "house call," "attitude," "isolation," and so on produces what I would call a ragtag bundle of articles. Most of them are descriptive—that is, the kind of research that tells us characteristics of populations. That research tells us that yes, most people like to be visited, and oh yes, when we visit old people at home we find all sorts of problems that nobody knew anything about. And I don't need to tell you what kind of problems those are: hypertension, osteoporosis, and so on. When authors try to do quantitative research (that is, the kind that allegedly establishes a cause and effect), the outcome is nearly always inconclusive. Where there *is* a conclusive study, there is usually another one to contradict it.

Descriptive research produces conclusions nobody ever doubted just based on common sense, and any kind of reasonable-quality quantitative research produces no conclusion whatsoever. Why do we bother?

Old people, with exceptions, generally hate loneliness and social isolation. What they want, I find, is freedom from this situation, on *their* terms. Quite often the kind of flexible social skills that an ordinary middle-aged working person or parent deploys every day just aren't there anymore, or the old person doesn't have the energy or the interest to deploy them. Not only are socially isolated old people all different from one another, they are often *very* different from one another, unpredictable, and quite fixed in their attitudes toward all sorts of things. What should we be doing for them, then? Would it occur to us to ask them what they want and then, if they do want our help, try to get it for them in a reasonably sensible way that respects their quirks?

We can add "not wanting to be painfully lonely and isolated" to our list of desires of fragile old people, but let's be sure to add to that "not wanting to be patronized" and "needing to design their own social interventions." Nobody would suggest that old people with collapsing capabilities can organize this kind of thing without help. But we'd better ask what they want first, and then custom design the program with the user in mind, if we want it to work.

We can generalize about what fragile elderly people want, but those conclusions are subject to heterogeneity. As I write this, I am preparing to do some descriptive research of my own, prompted by Dr. Davenport. My question is, How many people feel the way she does? How many fragile elderly people would prefer not to wake up in the morning?

In doing this descriptive research, I am not deluded enough to think that I will gain any better understanding of the frail elderly in general. What I'm hoping for is a bit better understanding of thirty or forty particular individuals.

But why do some people prefer not to experience the future? What would it take for them to want to wake up in the morning, to have Mr. Schoenfeld's idea that there might just be something interesting around the corner? If we were somehow able to keep from people a few of the things they *don't* want, it might make a difference. It may turn out that the most important reason to continue to get up in the morning is the kind of meaningful relationship Elzbieta Kalinska enjoys.

To summarize, what the fragile elderly *don't* want includes, first, being a burden. Many patients may not be able to appreciate that they are a burden, because of dementia or because they've just never been the kind of person who worries about anybody else. But most old people feel this sharply and are unable to avoid it. Like being near the end of life, having physical problems (or mental ones) that ordinary people find disgusting is something we really prefer not to talk about. How awful for a brilliant, proud, sophisticated person like Ann Davenport to see her daughter steel herself as she deals with a filthy-smelling mess on the floor. I am disgusting, is what's in that lady's mind.

But we need to recognize that incontinence, awful wounds, and offensive behavior do make people a burden, and we are dishonest with ourselves and our patients and loved ones when we don't admit this. There's a much better way to prevent people from hating themselves because of what we have to do for them, which will be discussed in the next chapter.

Second, the fragile elderly do not want to suffer. Both Maggie Dunlop and Emily Martin suffer from pain that we can only partly help. Health care as we practice it, at its very best, can't control everybody's symptoms. But it is important to get the cards on the table: suffering is real, we can't always make it go away, and it can be bad enough to make people want to die.

An old person in misery from pain, breathlessness, itching, or anything else that is hard to make better usually doesn't have much else on her mind. No difficulty figuring out what this person wants. And like not being a burden, not suffering intolerable symptoms is something we want for everyone but can't always get. But we can certainly continue trying.

Third, fragile old people don't want to be treated as a non-person. I used the hospital, one of my favorite demons, as an example of a situation where people are sometimes dehumanized. Treated as if they're not there. But this can happen in a nursing home, an apartment, or someone's house—wherever a caregiver is burnt out or in some other way frustrated in accomplishing what needs to be done to look after someone properly. When a patient is hateful to you—that is, when you hate what you have to do, or what you can't do, for him—it may just seem better to say nothing than to express yourself. It might seem kind, in a way, just to get it over with: go about your business and then go read a magazine or watch TV in the other room.

But old people who suspect, rightly or wrongly, that they are a burden will feel their suspicion confirmed if we treat them like a bed to be made. We'll explore solutions to this awful dilemma shortly; it's enough to say here that this is another general need among the fragile elderly: to be treated as a self.

Finally, maybe the most difficult need of all to meet is the need to not be painfully socially isolated, a need that has to be met in a way that works for each individual old person. And that includes some very fussy, rigid, "difficult" old people. Some of them have developed push-pull methods of dealing with attempts to help them, possibly out of bitter experience, possibly just because that's the way they are.

From the things old people want and need to avoid, the two positive wants emerge. Nearly all of my old patients are saying to me and to all of us, sometimes silently, "Please listen to me," and, "Please be with me."

How do we reinvent health care in the light of these wants and needs? Is there a way to take the traditional and modern priorities of prevention and rescue and reorient them so that they work for these people?

Chapter 10 discusses a fundamental change in approach, based on a change in attitude. The good news is that the change has already started. Not so good is how big and against the grain the change really needs to be. I imagine that we will end up getting the health care we deserve. When someone is looking to be heard, and for us to *be there*, an absent, proxy, or formulaic response will not do. Nothing will change until we do.

# 10 Starting Back
## Healthier Health Care

**CHUCK DAVIDSON**

A guy I used to play hockey with called: he and his siblings were having problems with Dad. I met the three adult kids at one of their nice upscale homes, and everybody greeted me in the living room, including old Chuck, who gave me a charming sideways smile as he shook my hand. He had on a button-down plaid shirt, cords, and a tennis hat.

One of the boys, now middle-aged and bald, started out, "Well, I'll just lay it out for you, John. Dad seems to be having problems getting things done. I keep getting calls, and I'm worried about getting that call I won't know how to handle." He looked around at his brother and sister, who nodded agreement. Chuck, for his part, would like to know exactly what kind of problems he was supposed to be having. All the kids responded to this with, "We just want what's best for you, Dad."

After everybody said his or her piece, I told them I can see that they all loved and cared about one another, but if the cards are really on the table, the kids had their own lives and were afraid that there was going to be an impossible-to-handle disaster involving Dad at exactly the wrong time. Dad said he knew that he wasn't going to live forever, but he was determined to make the best of whatever time he had left. Plus one thing he had always hated was being told what to do. Probably what you need to do, I told them, is have a few sessions sitting down together, talk about some practical things in the future, and see if you can be really honest with one another about what everybody needs. Then, I said, we could get together again and see if we can make some practical plans.

They all nodded their heads with studied interest as I made my little speech. Then the same middle-aged son said, "What are you going to do if you fall and hurt yourself, Dad? You know we just want what's best for you." Dad responded by accusing them of wanting to shut him up in a nursing home. And so on.

People talking without listening, as the song goes.

### HELEN ARNESEN

I get called sometimes to evaluate an old person's mental capability for things like whether they can manage their finances. A lawyer asked me to see a seventy-seven-year-old lady who had given her thirty-year-old boyfriend some expensive presents and looked to be about to change her will. The lawyer acted for the daughter.

I found my way at about 5 PM to the lady's address, which turned out to be a classy concrete-and-glass apartment building in a quiet neighborhood. It was obvious when Mrs. Arnesen answered the door that she had been drinking. She was expensively dressed, but her hair was a mess and her blouse wasn't buttoned correctly. She offered me a gin and tonic, as if I had arrived at a cocktail party. My mental status examination, in the clinical language of my report, described her as disinhibited and inappropriately seductive. No way could she coherently tell me anything about her finances, and she gave a gushing and glowing description of her boyfriend.

The lawyer, worried, I think, that his client's claim about her mother's incapability might be weakened by the fact that the mother was drunk, sent me back to see her again, this time at 10 AM. What a difference! This woman was pale and shaky but reasonable, coherent, quite serious, and sober. She described to me her ambivalence about the younger boyfriend. She knew perfectly well, she said, that he was partly interested in her money. They had even discussed that. And she waved her hand in the air, lighting a cigarette, as she told me she understood exactly how that kind of relationship would appear to other people. "But it isn't that simple," she said. "And besides, it's *my* money, right?"

And the young boyfriend, who was at least apparently open about his motives, was looking after her. He did the shopping, he took her out for dinner, he drove her to the doctor, he cleaned the apartment. Some nights they slept together. Mrs. Arnesen had fixed him up with a sporty summer wardrobe for their cruise to Alaska. The daughter hadn't been to see her in six months and had never lifted a finger to help.

When the light turns green, you go. When the light turns red, you stop. But what do you do when the light turns blue, with orange and lavender spots?

SHEL SILVERSTEIN

## INDRJIT DHALLIWAL

This eighty-nine-year-old retired carpenter was a pillar of the Indo-Canadian community in his town. He had built their church practically singlehandedly when he was younger, and dozens of people sought his advice right up until a few years ago, when his memory started to slip.

It would be hard to imagine two more different people than his daughters Marilyn and Donna. Marilyn was the soul of laissez-faire. As her dad lost his mobility and began to suffer from obscure pains and intermittent trouble breathing, Marilyn's instructions to me were, "Keep him comfortable." Mr. Dhalliwal had had a good life and was always philosophical about dying, she explained. Donna had different expectations. Her Internet searches revealed that people with dementia sometimes have tumors or something else pressing on the brain. She was concerned that her father might have vitamin deficiencies. She believed that if he could only get to the sort of world-class clinic that existed in Los Angeles, they could find out what was wrong with him. You can imagine which of the two sisters I tended to agree with.

About 10:30 one night, Marilyn (normally the relaxed one) called, obviously upset. Dad was having a lot of trouble, breathing heavily, grasping at his chest, and moaning. She couldn't communicate with him. Her sister was on her way. I got in the car and was there in about fifteen minutes. My evaluation left me with no clear diagnosis, but my patient was in awful distress. It could have been a heart attack, a lung clot, pneumonia, pressure inside the chest from bleeding or air, or just pain from nerves, muscles, or bones. I couldn't tell, and I didn't have morphine with me to at least get him comfortable.

We called an ambulance. Donna insisted we must; Marilyn wanted me to do something to make him comfortable, but there was nothing I could do. Donna's face said, There! You're finally going to get him the care he needs! Marilyn and I both understood that this was one of those situations, in a reverse sort of way, where the rules don't apply. Of the two unacceptable possibilities, the horror of critical care, starting with the ambulance and emergency room but with relief, we hoped, was better than the horror of what was going on in his living room.

Within five minutes of the crew's arrival, morphine had made Mr. Dhalliwal 90 percent more comfortable, and he was kept that way through the first twenty-four hours in the hospital. He managed to survive the firemen, ambulance crew, police, emergency room, CT scan, specialist evaluations, re-referrals, oxygen, swallowing assessment, psychiatric evaluation, rehabilitation, and everything else. He came home eventually, and stayed there.

We're here for a good time (not a long time)
TROOPER

I'VE BEEN TALKING about a collision and its consequences. A medical system designed to manage future risk through multiple-drug treatment and to perform high-tech rescues is involved in a slow-motion crash with the fragile elderly. Neither of the participants can walk away from it in one piece. There are also factors that appear to remove the controls from the hands of the people who should be able to steer clear of some of the trouble. So how do we fix what's wrong?

The most important answer is not to control or discipline the drug industry, to beat various kinds of doctors (or any other health professionals) over the head, to fix the hospitals, or to reform the way we do health care administration. Most of the answer lies instead with family members, doctors, nurses, and home support workers. All of us.

Before beginning to try to help a fragile old person, most of us only vaguely appreciate what we're in for. It is trouble, and it's usually big trouble by most normal standards. And modern, traditional, scientific health care will make it worse. Only a fundamental and radical change of attitude can get us through it feeling as if we did the right things. We need courage to make care for our old loved ones work in a way that feels right and to carefully decide, one by one, what parts, if any, of scientific medical care are helpful and what parts are not.

We badly need a change of heart to straighten out how we care for the fragile elderly. But what does that change look like? Fundamentally, old people's needs are best met with our finest human instincts, not with technology. Their care falls into *our* hands, not someone else's. The implied responsibility is great, but it is limited. We can succeed if we tell ourselves the truth about what's on our minds and what's happening, listen to old people, treat them as individual human beings, accept that they are near the ends of their lives, and don't try to hide our mixed feelings about them and what we have to do for them.

To succeed at looking after individual old people and at the same time change the system for the better, we need to develop and encourage some new attitudes. One of those attitudes is insisting that care be placed in *our* hands. If we are serious about that, we have to understand a little bit about what caregiving means and how to make it work for everyone. It will never be easy; when we take care into our own hands, we are going to have something significant, something heavy, to carry around.

But we have help. When someone enters what I call fragility, we're headed into some rough water, so it's a good idea to know where the rocks are and to prepare ourselves to avoid them. And finding that out is a cooperative enterprise. We're not on our own, *usually.* Caregiving goes forward with the support and advice of providers: doctors, nurses, social workers, and others. And I will spend some time on the characteristics of a good provider so that at least you can recognize one and, I hope, find one.

Communication between caregivers and providers counts. But there is a more important communication: with the old person herself and with *yourself.* This is absolutely basic, whatever role you're playing.

You also have to get rid of the idea that somebody, some expert or some book, is going to tell you exactly *when* a different approach to health care for fragile old people is supposed to kick in. Chapter 1 describes the people we're talking about. But the definition of the kind of people who will be harmed, not helped, by the medical system is really individual. People exist who never trust authority, who thrive on swimming against the stream, and who have been defining their own world—lifestyle, politics, and health care—since they were kids. They take naturally to opposing the common wisdom.

At the other end of the scale some people just need, trust, respect, and value a fixed set of rules. If you are a caregiver, you will be considering these values and attitudes on behalf of someone else.

Where is the elderly person you are caring for on that individuality scale? Most people will decide that the traditional health care system doesn't work for them anymore somewhere around the time that an elderly person is homebound and needs help every day. But you must take the time to find out what everyone involved really thinks and get the best advice you can from professional people you trust. There must eventually come a time when you cross a line and the priority is no longer prevention and rescue. But bottom line: you decide when that is. There is no reliable scientific medical rule to make that decision for you.

You should feel empowered to make that decision. Once you make it, it's time to start understanding that looking after your loved one is a human activity instead of a technical activity. But what does that mean?

Number one, it means responsibility. If you are doing the care and making the decisions, you are responsible. But you share that responsibility with everybody who's helping you: family members, home support people, the doctors and nurses. But the flip side is that that responsibility is usually surprisingly light. It is comfort and function we're responsible for, not some complicated technical cardiac output or glandular performance measured by experts and machines. Those who are closest to an old person regularly are in the best position to understand and see to comfort and function. Much of what needs to be done is best understood instinctively, not by measurement with a scientific instrument.

Doing things for a complicated older person may not be simple or easy, though. And it changes from time to time. Some people may decide to pay someone else to help if it is impossible to do it all by themselves. But it will work best, and most likely avoid the clutches of completely inappropriate formulaic health care, if we take responsibility for it back to ourselves and quit contracting out decisions and planning. There are always exceptions. Some older people have no family and no resources. There are many halfway measures, including paying for shopping, errands, meals, and personal care. This depends on your resources. It can happen that institutional care is the only option.

Sometimes it is impossible to give direct care because you live far away. In this situation paying for care or using (possibly partly using) an institutional system may be the best that can be done. But a world of difference exists between having advocating, supportive close relatives that one can call on and who visit regularly, and having nobody at all, or relatives who default to routine medical care by experts and hospitals.

You don't have to go back to university or read a dozen how-to manuals on caregiving to be responsible. It has its technical side, but normally a caregiver is not directly responsible for that. The *medical* part of caregiving is very well within the capability of an ordinary family doctor and can usually be done at home. What kind of dressings or laxatives to use, whether a walker is appropriate or not, and how many hours of home care are needed are the business of good primary care nurses, physiotherapists, and social workers.

People understand, and assume, responsibility in different ways. Take the Dhalliwal sisters, for instance. Laid-back Marilyn was comfortable with broad philosophical decision making but wasn't much of a housekeeper. Detail-oriented Donna, an accountant, could handle an endless pile of whatever kind of detail as long as it didn't contain anything abstract. Although I lean toward Marilyn's approach, details are also important.

So the first thing to do after deciding to get rid of a prevention-and-rescue approach to care is to get responsibility for an old person into your own hands, away from the experts and out of institutions. Make no mistake: experts and institutions equal prevention and rescue in today's health care system. What we want is no drugs that don't make the person feel better and no hospital unless there is a clear goal that can't be met any other way. Just *decide*, and then stick to that decision as much as possible.

One of the toughest of the responsibilities we face as supporters or caregivers is also another important attitude that we need: honesty. This is not always an easy burden to bear. But you can't do human—as opposed to technical—care without it.

I'm not talking about honesty as some sort of Platonic virtue but as a practical necessity to get the job done. The core idea is similar to the one expressed by Ivan Illich at the beginning of Chapter 8. Modern medical care operates according to a formula, and while that formula may be true in some abstract sense, it is a million miles from the *whole truth* about an elderly person. Telling all of the truth includes admitting limitations and mistakes. Something went wrong, I think it was my fault, I feel bad about it, now let's get busy and see if we can fix it. This is bound up, of course, with taking responsibility. But be honest. Ignoring difficult or awkward facts or feelings will stop caregiving in its tracks faster than just about anything else. That goes for doctors and caregivers equally.

The Davidson family is at the start of their journey toward honesty. The dad is fine, for the moment. But the kids quite correctly see caregiving on the near horizon, and they don't like the look of it. I hope they will start telling one another and their father what's really on their minds, but if they don't, the old man is in for repeated trips to the hospital, early nursing home admission, and probably some bewildered, bitter disillusionment. I sense another example of the acorn falling not far from the tree.

Taking a human approach to looking after old people like the ones I see at their homes also involves respect for individuality. Expecting an old person to be like anybody else is a recipe for conflict and unhappiness. Difficult conversations can be impossible if as caregivers and providers we have a two-dimensional picture of what somebody old and frail is like. A daughter might remember her mom from the last time the two really spent any time with one another. Four decades ago. But now the mum is in a completely different world. Forget the old issues and look realistically at what's in front of you.

In thinking about diagnosis and treatment, a doctor must also recognize the individuality of his patient. The doctor who will keep someone out of the hospital is the one who sees her patient as a self.

The worst thing that can happen to a fragile old person is to go to the hospital *unless* they are Mr. Dhalliwal the night I saw him at home. The three rules about rules for the fragile elderly are exception, exception, and exception. You can't fix a broken hip in someone's living room.

I talked with a very old lady not long ago after we had swatted our way through a perfunctory medical visit at her home. This woman I knew to have been a stunning beauty when she was younger. It took some imagination to see how that could have been, looking at her now, but I could still feel the magnetism of her personality. We talked about the changes of aging, and she said to me, "Doctor, I had no idea things were going to turn out this way. You can't imagine what it feels like to be like (she gestured eloquently toward herself) *this*."

When we look at an elderly person in need of help as something abstract, the help we provide will be effete—ineffective. When we see the person, listen to their wants and needs, and understand just how unique, how *strange*, their experience really is, we start to build a basis for doing something creative and real for them. These people are, as we all will be, who and what they are, and they don't normally have the energy or time to pretend otherwise. Respect that individuality, warts and all.

The human side of care also involves accepting things we can't change (and having "the wisdom to know the difference"). All my patients really are near the end of life. Nobody knows *how* near, but still, relatively speaking, it is near. But caregivers often do not understand that though they are responsible for seeing that their old relative's remaining life is a good time, it's *not* a long time. It's okay, I would say, to enjoy the positive aspect of that ambivalence.

The medical system's priorities are prevention and rescue. Much of this book is about what a bad idea those priorities, as we usually practice them, are for the fragile elderly. But could we reorient prevention and rescue somehow? Is there some good we can squeeze out of all these perfectly natural and reasonable ideas? I think so.

Rescue implies a crisis. Crisis for a fragile old person is a crisis of function. The proper rescue is to support function. But there are exceptions, like Mr. Dhalliwal. There are times when only the hospital can give you what you need, and it would be awful for me to be misunderstood to be uncompromising about not going to the hospital. But for goodness' sake, if you are lucky enough to have a primary care medical person (family doctor, that is) who knows the elderly patient and understands her priorities, never send such a patient into an emergency room without a phone call from that doctor to put the receiving professionals in the picture. The first response to crisis is always, though, support of function and comfort. *Then* you can start worrying about fixing what's wrong.

I don't understand what we are trying to prevent in elderly people near the end of their lives, especially with the usual drug-based preventive care. But there is prevention with a more human face than prolonging life and preventing diseases that someone already has. That prevention is individual, and it will be effective only as long as we, the ones closest to the old person, are personally involved in making sure the prevention meets the commonsense test.

Earlier I talked about what elderly people want and need to *avoid:* being a burden to those who love them, suffering incurable symptoms, being treated like an object, and being isolated and lonely. Can we prevent these things old people fear and would love to not experience?

Not wishing to be a burden on someone we love is complicated. If we are an elderly person, wouldn't someone like our son or grandchild (who presumably loves us too) be quite happy to help? Isn't it a convoluted kind of blame we direct at them when we presume they don't like looking after us? What, really, is the limit of what they will do for us happily and willingly?

This is where honesty comes in. I've seen genuinely well-intentioned people who love and respect one another getting to the point where, when all the cards are on the table, the old person still feels guilty and as though they are imposing. The only preventive remedy for this kind of thing is a statement by the caregivers that their love is *unconditional.* Mum, you did it for me. And someone else will do it for me again at the end of my life. But even without that, I'm doing it and will continue because I love you.

Two of my patients described in the last chapter suffered from intolerable pain that we couldn't do enough about. I could have told symptom-control stories with a little happier ending, and there are lots of these. Using the methods learned from palliative care and from the new discipline of pain medicine, and with our knowledge of drugs and biology, we really can do a lot to prevent pain and other distressing symptoms these days if we are committed to success and if we individualize the treatment. This is an important part of the doctor's job.

Prevention makes sense when we talk about pain. One of the principles of pain control is to give enough medication that pain doesn't happen at all. We treat the ugly expectation of pain by preventing the pain. There are doctors who still worry about narcotic addiction in people who are in pain. But addiction or dependence is likelier if we *don't* control pain well enough. And whether the symptom is pain, breathlessness, nausea, or drowsiness, we have the advantage that we know when we have succeeded: the symptom is better! That knowledge is worth an awful lot more than an abstract promise that some event in the future maybe, relatively speaking, for some people, in an ideal world, is not going to happen.

Pain and other symptoms, are not just disturbing by themselves; they can also make someone start to feel hopeless. And a hopeless, depressed person feels symptoms more sharply. That vicious cycle can be broken: even if the pain doesn't go away completely, we can attack and prevent depression and hopelessness directly, with drugs or with comforting touch or conversation.

We can't control every distressing symptom. But we can make nearly all of them a lot better. We can certainly try, and we *must* try—and keep trying. Preventing pain and other symptoms is a big priority. As caregivers, insist on that doggedness. Don't let your doctors and nurses off the hook!

I don't know what the solution is for bad hospital care. The best thing to do is keep fragile old people away. That works for me because most of my patients, most of the time, can't benefit from what is done best in the hospital: single-disease cure and rescue. And even if some potential benefit existed, the disastrous social and physical results of enforced bed rest and bewildering, futile investigation and care might not be worth it. If you don't want your loved one to be treated like an object, keep him at home if you can, with people he knows and trusts.

And if your family member does go into the hospital, work hard at getting her out. Make sure somebody who knows and who cares about her sees her every single day. Don't fall into the trap of believing everything you are told in the hospital. Get the help of your informed family doctor. If days and days go by with nothing appearing to happen, if you can't get hold of anybody on the phone to explain things, or if you can't understand why an old person wouldn't be better off at home, make a fuss. If you can be reasonably sure (and, again, this usually involves the collaboration of an informed family physician or home care nurse at a minimum) that care can proceed at home, carefully consider discharge from the hospital against medical advice. I realize this is heresy, but I have to say it. Preventing the hospital catastrophe is worth bending a few rules.

People who are lonely and who really want companionship can be prevented from being isolated and feeling hopeless if we can find, as we did for Frank Hamaguchi in Chapter 9, some arrangement that suits them for getting together with other people. But we have to make sure we don't make things worse. Becoming old increases people's suspicion about being patronized, with some justification. The best solution is to listen carefully and try to hear what an old person needs. They may not tell you in so many words.

A good friend, a retired nurse who visits the elderly at home as a volunteer, warns me that when a visit fails, it's because we don't ask the old person's agenda. She used to visit in the hospital and see people the night before surgery. The topic of conversation was *never* the surgery. Politics, cooking, life in the North, raising kids. The secret is to let the person you're visiting set the topic.

Taking responsibility ourselves, telling the truth, recognizing individual differences, finding our way to comfort about life's end, and giving care that focuses on what our old patients and loved ones want and need is not going to happen overnight. But I'm starting to see the change beginning around me in small ways. Doctors and teams of professionals exist who are dedicated to home care and whose practices and attitudes are calculated to meet old people's needs. I'm beginning to see softening of the rules regarding admission in some enlightened emergency rooms.

There is no hidden agenda. If you believe that keeping an old lady away from the hospital is a violation of her fundamental rights, or a way to save money, then it wouldn't surprise me if you objected to my ideas about keeping her at home. The same applies to cutting down on the number of drugs people like my patients take. Only a hypocrite would try to deny that good humane care of fragile old people is going to save resources. That's what Chapter 7 was all about: the system can't stand the strain, either.

But the important reason to not practice traditional prevention and rescue on people like Mary McCarthy is that they are bad for *her*. Preventing harm to the health care system is a secondary benefit. The standard of care I'm advocating is different from, not less than, what we accept as best practice now. I think we'll get there.

Both caregivers and care providers must be committed. That means that what happens needs to *matter* to each individual person. We're making progress when we start thinking of the people caring for an old person by name, with lives and families of their own, not generically as her family, her providers, or her home support agency.

I'm going to describe caregiving and care providing as I think they should look, keeping in mind that neither one is possible without the other.

Most of us don't come to caregiving as a chosen profession. Caregivers don't walk up to the door with a photo-ID card and a black bag full of dressings and brochures. We fall sideways into it when our parent, husband or wife, friend, or neighbor needs us. And it tends to defy the how-to manuals' descriptions. It's messy.

And not just the physical business of cleaning someone who can't clean themselves, but also our relationship with them and the struggles we may have with the extent of our responsibility. But I have a life. Mum was always stingy; now I'm expected to pay for everything. Donald was the most selfish bastard in the world; now he's helpless and I'm supposed to love feeding him? I didn't ask to be the one to make Mrs. Lopez's dinner; where the hell is her son? Remember, for the elderly person, better the struggles and ambivalence than the hospital or nursing home. They're here for a good time, not a long time.

Dealing with these feelings isn't easy, and I know of no formula that works in every situation. Although there is no substitute for honesty, some situations can't fully survive it. There is no benefit in telling someone whose memory is very impaired all about your ambivalence and concerns, only to have to repeat yourself any number of times. If instinct tells you that now is not the time to start pushing sensitive buttons, it may be better to wait. Or even never to push the buttons at all.

Caregiving is work. And if the caregiver is a family member, usually it is work done for free and for somebody with whom you already have a complicated relationship. What does the old person really want and need? What is the caregiver offering? What are her obligations? What are the limits? What do we do when we get to that limit?

It would be rare for a caregiver to ask, or even think of, these terribly important questions until she is up to her eyeballs in the daily grind. But one of the most difficult parts of caregiving is tied up with the answers to those questions.

Caregivers come in all shapes and sizes, and they have their own needs. They may be male or female, young or old, more or less willing, assertive or shy, informed or not, able or troubled with health care problems themselves. I've never met a perfect caregiver. The vignette about Helen Arnesen illustrates that flawed or unconventional caregiving may be all that's available. It is absolutely better than nothing where nothing leads to the default of the hospital or a nursing home. The broadest of possible minds is needed in deciding who is an adequate caregiver where it's really needed and who isn't. Mrs. Arnesen's boyfriend was making a trade. Its exact terms may not be to everyone's taste. But there is, needs to be, something in the arrangement for caregivers.

It may be meeting a sense of duty. But people often feel trapped by caregiving. Someone might just find it unthinkable not to look after someone, for example, especially a close family member, and especially if there's no one else to do it. But the role of caregiver tends to be a short piece. Which for some people can be the silver lining of the cloud they find themselves under looking after someone else. And it isn't, or shouldn't be, a solo performance.

The caregiving relationship is subject to some unexpected dynamics. A domineering spouse is now helpless. The brainier partner in a relationship is now demented. Someone dearly loved for a generation drifts into abusive behavior. Old conflicts, suppressed or never really understood, erupt. With worsening memory impairment, hope for resolving old issues fades. But opportunities to succeed exist in the face of all this complexity.

The task of caregiving lives on information. And information is available. Ask questions! Find other people in a similar situation and ask them how they manage. Find a caregivers' support group and go to some of the meetings. Inquire about respite. Get on the computer or the telephone and see what books, agencies, and programs are out there. Wasting huge amounts of effort on things that can be done easily, or just failing to use strategies everyone knows about, is tragic and preventable.

Get help. Sharing the burden is preferable to acute or chronic institutional care, which is the completely inadequate "safety net" under failed caregiving.

Many caregivers are, or see themselves as, unassertive. Getting what you want and need to get the job done may mean developing some new skills to go along with your new attitudes. If you find after trying that you just can't, for example, seem to get a case manager or a doctor to *hear* you, you may need—literally or otherwise—to speak louder. Getting help may involve finding someone who is naturally more able to make demands of others.

Many caregivers are so dedicated to their task that they suffer themselves. Burning out by taking on too much may seem hard to avoid, but success at helping someone else depends on sustaining yourself. Supporting the supporters should be a priority for us health professionals, but if it isn't, you may have to support yourself. This is another very important kind of honesty. I've seen many wonderful helpers drive themselves to the point of physical or emotional exhaustion pretending they're superhuman. Much as we might admire people for that sort of dedication, if you really want to keep an old person in his home and see to his needs, letting yourself burn out as a caregiver just isn't smart. You are part of the vital equipment.

This may mean compromise. Like the trades made by people like Helen Arnesen, you as a caregiver may have to change your rules a little. Let someone else take over for a while. Accept less than perfect performance from yourself. Relax! Get away, and not just for a few hours.

Unfortunately, not everyone *has* a caregiver. In an ideally supported world, we would provide one. Even where paid caregivers are available and funded, it's very hard to replace someone who has known an elderly person for a long time and has a personal stake in their well-being. Sadly, nursing homes tend to contain many people who are just alone in the world.

Good caregiving happens in some surprising circumstances. I've seen wonderful contented and balanced arrangements where caregivers have no personal relationship with the elderly person, in physically awful living situations, and under fairly extreme compromise. But however it happens, a good caregiver will tend to find good care providers, and good providers encourage and support good caregiving. A good deal all around.

Providers are the professionals. In my community we are beginning to see changes that reflect the attitudes I advocate. More doctors are seeing people at home. Groups of professionals are cooperating and really communicating with one another. Agency policies and procedures are beginning to allow exceptions to such things as professional role boundaries and "safety." A doctor working in a team, for example, might delegate checking on a patient's walking (after he starts a potentially dangerous medicine) to a physiotherapist. The physiotherapist might trust a nurse to help somebody with her walker. Progress! But we have a way to go.

A health care professional who understands what you want and need, and whom you trust, can make all the difference to the success of your caregiving. Following is a description of the preferred pattern of professional care for the fragile elderly, focusing on medical care, particularly general practice, family practice, or primary care. I hope it will give you an idea what kind of people you'll probably find it easiest to work with.

Medical care of fragile homebound people is care at home. Period. A visit to a doctor's office by a frail elderly person simply doesn't work. Although dragging that person into a family practice office is less likely to result in futile dangerous medical care than taking the same person to a hospital, the office is designed for a completely different kind of medical experience. Doctors and other professionals need to get on the road and see their elderly patients at home.

Good medical care of homebound people is primary care. The model of medical care in which a generalist refers clinical problems to specialists is also unworkable with the fragile elderly. Specialists don't see people at home. As a forty-year-old, you may have a digestive problem, go and see a digestive specialist, take medication or have some kind of a procedure done, and that's that. But the multiply pathological fragile elderly have problems that can never be solved in that way, and they have all sorts of them, potentially involving a dozen specialists.

Remembering Henri Boisvert, the noisy nursing home patient in Chapter 6, we appreciate that an old person with those kinds of problems needs detailed care but can also get into a lot of preventable trouble without a doctor who is watching the overall picture. A style of medical care where problems are understood to be *concluded* by referral to a specialist or by a piece of technical information is upside down for my people. And dangerous.

What's good about primary care is also what's bad about it: you're stuck with people for the longer haul. Telling someone that their problem is not in my area of expertise doesn't end the transaction or my responsibility. I feel at times as if I'm riding alongside my patients on a very bumpy road. I'm not in the same vehicle with them, but we do share the potholes. The better I get to know them, the more absurd the usual single-system or single-disease approaches that work for people with one problem appear. Insist on real primary care. Forget specialists.

But because the fragile elderly have an unpredictable response to medication, we don't know what is going to happen when a drug is given to them. Every prescription is an experiment. And the essence of experiment is observation: what happened? The answer determines what to do next. It is not safe or reasonable to do any other kind of prescribing for the fragile elderly.

Doctors sometimes call this pattern of drug prescription the "$n = 1$" clinical trial, $n$ being the symbol for the sample size in drug trials. Thus, $n = 1$ means this drug trial has only one subject. The subject is *somebody* who gets the drug, and then something happens (or not). Because in an $n = 1$ trial, something actually happens to an individual rather than to a large group, and we can see what that is, if our eyes are open. With a preventive drug, it is impossible ever to tell whether an event you are taking medicine to prevent in the future would or would not have happened if you had *not* taken the drug; so you can't do an $n = 1$ trial of prevention.

These $n = 1$ trials depend on measurable outcomes. The logic here is inescapable, and the conclusion is that frail older people shouldn't normally be taking drugs for prevention.

Again, I have some problems with the generality of epidemiology. It isn't clearly scientific, in that it isn't easily falsifiable. Most important to the oddball black swans in a population, the conclusions of modern medicine, based in epidemiology, don't promise anything specifically to an individual. So things didn't go well? Obviously you weren't part of the group. But when the group has a population of one, there's no such escape. Reference to the "group" is easy: it's *you!*

Let's say that a ninety-one-year-old Mr. Hasim is breathless. After examining him, I decide I can probably get him to feel better by giving him some more heart failure treatment. My hypothesis, or scientific rule, about this particular situation is that he's having trouble breathing because he's in heart failure and that heart failure treatment will improve his breathing. *It's falsifiable.* If after two days on extra heart failure medicine he's no better, my hypothesis is junk. I try something else. And if the population is just this particular old man, nobody else, he is the white swan, the black swan, and also the blue one with orange and lavender spots. This is the science that works for the fragile elderly and the kind that leads to the safest regimen of drugs. And it is rigorous and true to the scientific method.

Prescribing for old people is trial and error; it's as simple as that. Except sometimes it's not so simple. Recently I gave an eighty-eight-year-old woman a medication for arthritis because she was in pain whenever she tried to walk and so had quit walking. A week later I came back to see what had happened. The picture was gray, not black or white. The pain was a bit better, *probably,* but now she had heartburn, which meant she had trouble sleeping, which meant she was tired most of the day, which meant she was walking even less. Function doesn't always improve the way we expect.

Another patient, an old gentleman in assisted living, first came to me on twelve medications, fresh out of the hospital. A male Mary McCarthy, except he wasn't in nearly as bad shape. On the principle that less is better, and based on my skeptical attitude about hospital doctors' prescribing, I started reducing the dose of a couple of drugs that lower blood pressure. To make a long story short, this gentleman actually had more heart trouble when his blood pressure was high (this is rare, but it happens). He had the kind of heart failure that occurs because the heart is not able to pump against high pressure, so lowering his blood pressure was good for him, and letting it rise made him quite short of breath. Less medication isn't always better.

All very interesting. But how, as someone who is not medically trained, are you supposed to know if a doctor is prescribing in a reasonable way? Here are a few hints.

Is the doctor talking about drugs to make the old person feel better and function better? If not, if the doctor is talking about medication for prevention—for cholesterol, for blood pressure, or for osteoporosis—you may want to think twice. Does the doctor come back and check what's happened after starting, stopping, or changing a drug? Does she ask questions about how a person has been feeling since the drug change? Does she check to see whether the drug has helped or not? Your doctor should be interested in your observations about whether things have improved or gotten worse.

Is the doctor trying to keep the amount of medication reasonable? Does he seem to know what the old person is taking when he visits? Does he ask if the old person is taking the medication, ask to see the pill bottles, and even count the pills? Not only should doctors be worried about medication in old people, they should try to *stop* some of it. This has been called the "selective drugectomy," the removal of certain drugs. But after cutting down the dose or stopping some medicine, the doctor should have the same kind of vigilant, thorough concern about the result as if he had started a new treatment.

If a doctor gives you the impression that she knows what's going to happen when she gives an old person medication, she's either got a very impressive bedside manner or she isn't doing her job properly. We want doctors to exude confidence and reassurance, but I'm much more reassured when the doctor is worried. Worried and being careful.

Choosing a doctor presents a few practical problems. They're human, and they tend to be different from one another in their attitude toward old people and the medical system. And it is a struggle for a doctor at this stage in history to strike out on her own, break the rules, and do the reasonable thing, the correct thing, with medicine instead of the preventive-guidelines thing. So you'll probably run into a range of different attitudes toward the kind of trial-and-error prescribing I'm advocating.

Also, in my community at least, family doctors are pretty hard to come by these days. Even harder to find is somebody who will come and see you at home. So it's all very well for me to tell you to go doctor shopping when there might not be an awful lot of merchandise on the shelves.

To make matters worse, not every family doctor is up to the challenge of home care of the elderly. I'm not trying to pretend it's rocket science, but there are usually several problems at once, quite a bit of medication, some psychological trouble, and all the business to do with the family, caregiving, the rest of the home care team, and so on. Decisions have to be deferred or made with limited information. Doctors, nurses, and other professionals who lack skills, can't handle decisions, don't know how to give reassurance when uncertain themselves, are inexperienced, or are looking for a holiday from demanding work should find some other kind of work to do. And you should steer clear of them if you can.

What if your family doctor, trusted and respected for decades, just doesn't look as if he or she is willing to "bend the rules," even if guidelines-style prescribing is making your relative worse? The important thing here is the *relationship*. If you find you can talk to the doctor, then you need to do that. If you can't, you might have to look for somebody else. Many doctors will respond to your patience and a little bit of gratitude (often they don't get a whole lot of either). Both of you are after the same outcome. Before you leave a long-trusted practitioner, make sure there's no hope of changing his mind.

That's the bottom line with providers: the relationship. It would be wonderful if every pharmacist, physiotherapist, doctor, and nurse were both a wonderful, warm-hearted helper and a computer-like technocrat. But given the choice, I think we're better off with people we feel we can trust.

All the trusted help in the world doesn't quite accomplish what we need, however. Most important to honest and humane care of fragile old people are the difficult conversations we must have. The fundamental idea behind caregiving is a sort of contract you make with the person you are caring for. Again, honesty is essential. And the contract, often, is really with yourself. As with providers, it's the relationship that matters, but the relationship can be much more stressful and complicated than the one you have with your nurse or nutritionist. This is the crux of making bad, overly technical care go away. It's where all the good attitudes come together to make things work.

There are two types of difficult conversations. First, you have to discuss advance directives, the decisions you make in advance about what you're going to do in certain kinds of future situations. Once you have made these decisions, they will express your idea that conventional care doesn't make sense for someone old and fragile. Second, you have to discuss your responsibility as a caregiver, and that one is a little harder to deal with, because you have to define, maybe redefine, the relationship.

In talking about advance directives, older people and their families need to think carefully, and speak honestly to one another, about how important the beliefs behind conventional health care are to them. What is an old person willing to go through, and how badly does she want to prolong life, honestly? What am I supposed to do when the traditional panic situations like shortness of breath or chest pain occur? Usually, the moment these questions are asked, differences of opinion arise, and emotions start to be involved. Putting our expectations into words is sometimes painful. Some people have a lot of trouble just talking about dying at home, for example. But once the ice is broken, it is usually surprising how quickly secretly held opinions can be shared. "One thing I can tell you for sure: I'll die before I go back to that hospital!"

Advance directives should be written down, and they should include certain likely scenarios. Do you want to go to the hospital? In what situations do you imagine you would want to go to the hospital? For me, the two most important questions are, Which is more important to you, prolonging life or staying comfortable? and, Who do you want to make decisions for you if you can't decide for yourself? Those two would be my version of bare-bones advance directives. They can include a little more information than that, but they are your decision in writing to give humane rather than technical care.

Sometimes the best advance directives come from an understanding of *attitudes,* and often these are remembered but don't get written down. How, really, do you feel about dying? Honestly now, what are you most afraid of? But the questions must be asked if you want to know the answer.

I don't think elderly people and their caregivers can understand one another on the subject of care without getting its "burden" out on the table. This may be the hardest part. And it can be even more difficult if the old person you're caring for can't participate. Then the conversation is going to be with *yourself.* But, more than anything, it's fear of trying to achieve this kind of understanding, along with fear of too great a burden, that drives people in the direction of useless rescue and prevention.

The big question is, What am I responsible for? How much do I have to do, really? This discussion can be exquisitely sensitive because elderly people are afraid of being a burden, and adult children or others can imagine getting stuck in an awful conflict between performing a very difficult task and having a life.

Talk about it!

Whether you are struggling with your own conscience or having a conversation with someone you will be helping, the relationship between the helper and the helped needs its personal responsibilities defined and *limited.*

Somehow, without getting into an argument and without either of you falsely denying your own needs, you must come to some kind of agreement: a contract. There are many questions, and their answers matter. How many hours is it safe to leave you alone? When is it okay to bring somebody in to help? What does "clean" mean (to you, to me, to my wife, to the home care nurse)? You think I like changing your diaper? Thing is, you changed mine! What about going to a nursing home?

This contract or understanding will change over time. But it needs to be clear so that the older person can rely on it and so that the caregiver understands where responsibility begins and ends. But the need for clarity, and its final achievement, is driven by how the two people feel about one another.

When my kids were little, I would from time to time read them *Love You Forever,* by Robert Munsch. The story is of a young woman who has a child, cares for him, and sees her baby grow up to be a man. All through the years she repeats to her boy, "I'll love you forever, I'll like you for always, as long as I'm living my baby you'll be." The young woman gets older and then becomes fragile. And toward the end of the story it's the son who cares for his mother and repeats exactly the same reassurance his mother used to give him. I was never able to finish that story without tears in my eyes, which I'm sure left my own children wondering what was the matter with Dad.

That sentiment is the one that makes caring for old people work. And no matter how difficult or conflicted the caregiving contract conversation, in the end the old person, now helpless, relies on our honoring the very old and fundamentally human obligation that's implied by our having grown up and been cared for.

So caregiving isn't a scientific or technical creature. When things are awkward and we need to know how we're doing, there really isn't a scientific answer to the question. Difficult as it may seem when we're used to trusting scientific thinking, *how something feels* is the most reliable measure of success at this enterprise. This operates in simple ways (I'm hot, I'm cold, I'm wet, I'm scared, I'm happy) or more complicated ones (you give me confidence, I don't trust him, I need to be left alone, I think I finally understand).

Trust the expression you see on the face, not the blood pressure. Trust your intuition, not your calculation. Think about what you're doing, but in the end, trust your heart, not your mind.

Your responsibility to an old person will end, probably sooner rather than later, but how you feel about what you did and didn't do will last a long, long time.

## Epilogue

When I visited Mrs. McCarthy after she got out of the hospital, my feelings as I walked over to her were not happy or very hopeful. I interrupted the story to tell you about old people and the medical system, and here we are back in Mary's dark living room. I'll pick up where I left off.

HER RESPONSES TO my questions didn't mean much. She seemed to be somewhere else, mumbling about her husband (long dead) and then falling asleep. She was pale, shaky, and a bit stiff. I got my tools out and examined her: her breathing was okay, but she had a very fast heartbeat and very low blood pressure.

In the list of medication, I could see drugs I knew were part of the guidelines for treating all of the "diseases" that her daughter, Gwen, had mentioned. Among them were six that lower blood pressure, with potentially harmful results. Another four or five could be biologically harmful in other ways. It may seem strange, but to me this was good news: something I might be able to fix!

Gwen and I agreed that we wanted to try to get Mary better at home, even if there was some risk she could die. Gwen believed that Mary would rather die than go back to the hospital. Gwen was willing to stay for a couple of days, but she would have to go to work eventually. She had called a home nursing agency, and someone was coming in to have a look at Mary McCarthy the next day.

MARY MCCARTHY RESPONDED to my selective drugectomy. Her blood tests showed mineral abnormalities, which I knew were coming from some of the medication. I kept carefully making drug changes and watching the results. In two weeks she was walking around her main floor, talking nearly normally, and eating and drinking without help. You can imagine my relief, considering that it was my failing to visit her at home in the first place that got her into all of this trouble.

She never got back to driving her car, but she still made it to the bridge club by taxi. Her grandchildren had mixed feelings about her starting up again with her sermons on work ethic, and I wasn't sure how I felt about arguing with her again, either. She and Gwen have had some serious conversations about what to do the next time she doesn't feel well. Gwen has come to understand that neither of them can escape personal responsibility for what happens to Mary.

On the bright side, Mary has had a visit from an older gentleman she met in the hospital, who also escaped and survived.

## Acknowledgments

I HESITATE TO implicate anyone in what may be received by many as a bad book. If you feel that way about it, I ask you to try to imagine what it would have been like if I had had to do it on my own.

Alan Cassels, a real author, called me one day with the idea of writing something about the elderly and their care, especially with drugs. The early outline of the book, and a lot of advice and information about writing in general, came from him. I wouldn't have done anything without his initial concept and introduction to the publishers. Years ago I got involved in discussions with Jonathan Berkowitz and then Ken Basset about problems with the medical system. This is as close as I could come, gentlemen, to the book we imagined writing.

Being a doctor, looking after old people, and eventually doing nothing but house calls was made possible by the teaching, mentoring, and encouragement of Peter Larkin, Bill Dalziel, Lyn Beattie, Bill McArthur, Helmut Ruebsaat, Harry Caine, Archie Johnson, Martha Donnelly, Ray Ancill, Larry Dian, Janet Martini, Chris Rauscher, Grady Meneilly, Mark Williams, Duncan Robertson, Judy Kelly, Laurel Chan, Sue Porter, Sam Sheps, Jamie Warren, Les Sheldon, Bob Rangno, Kieth Anderson, Rick Hudson,

Nigel Clark, Darryl Morris, John Feightner, Ian Schokking, Beverly Spring, David Brook, Will Johnston, Larry Barzelai, Shel Nathanson, Jay Slater, Ted Rosenberg, Mark Nowaczynski, Peter Grantham, Carol Herbert, and many, many others.

I've received encouragement and advice or ideas for the book (without their knowing it, in some cases) from Bob Rangno, Beverly Abercrombie, Joan McEwen, Sal Sloan, Robin Sloan, Peter Silin, Bob Kane, Fred Koning, Rick Hudson, and Bill Dalziel. Alister Brown and Gordon Sloan let me bounce philosophical ideas off them. Geoffrey Sloan provided solid moral support.

Somehow telephone conversations with Nancy Flight and Rob Sanders of Greystone Books gave only an inkling of what wonderful people they are in person. Nobody could ask for a gentler and more effective editor than Nancy. Their work is impeccable, but that's nothing beside their kindness, encouragement, and the risk they took in letting me get into print.

Thanks, and in some cases apologies, finally, to all the people and families of those who have been subject to my eccentric style of medical care. You've given me very much more than I could ever give you.

# References

**INTRODUCTION**

Best, J. *Damned Lies and Statistics*. Los Angeles: University of California Press, 2001.

Bird, A. *Philosophy of Science*. Montréal, Kingston, London, Buffalo: McGill-Queen's University Press, 1998.

Hazzard, W., et al., eds. *Principles of Geriatric Medicine and Gerontology*. 5th ed. New York: McGraw-Hill, 2003.

Rothman, K., ed. *Causal Inference*. Chestnut Hill, MA: Epidemiology Resources Inc., 1988.

Walker, A.M. *Observation and Inference: An Introduction to the Methods of Epidemiology*. Chestnut Hill, MA: Epidemiology Resources Inc., 1991.

**CHAPTER ONE**

Bergman, H., et al. "Frailty: An Emerging Research and Clinical Paradigm—Issues and Controversies." *Journals of Gerontology: Biological Sciences and Medical Sciences* 62 (2007): 731–37.

Ravaglia, G., et al. "Development of an Easy Prognostic Score for Frailty Outcomes in the Aged." *Age and Ageing* 37 (2008): 161–66.

Rockwood, K., and A. Mitnitski. "Frailty in Relation to the Accumulation of Deficits." *Journals of Gerontology: Biological Sciences and Medical Sciences* 62 (2007): 722–27.

Rockwood, K., et al. "A Global Clinical Measure of Fitness and Frailty in Elderly People." *Canadian Medical Association Journal* 173 (2005): 489–95.


**CHAPTER TWO**

Feyerabend, P. *Conquest of Abundance: A Tale of Abstraction vs. the Richness of Being.* Chicago: University of Chicago Press, 1999.

Hacking, I. *Representing and Intervening: Introductory Topics in the Philosophy of Natural Science.* Cambridge, U.K.: Cambridge University Press, 1983.

Hume, D. *An Enquiry Concerning Human Understanding.* 1748.

Popper, K. *The Logic of Scientific Discovery.* 1934. English edition. New York: Basic Books, 1959.

Rothman, K., ed. *Causal Inference.* Chestnut Hill, MA: Epidemiology Resources Inc., 1988.

Schulz, K., et al. "Empirical evidence of bias. Dimensions of Methodological Quality Associated with Estimates of Treatment Effects in Controlled Trials." *Journal of the American Medical Association* 273 (1995): 408–12.

Sibbald, B. "Understanding Controlled Trials: Why Are Randomised Controlled Trials Important?" *British Medical Journal* 316 (1998): 201.

Taleb, N. *Fooled by Randomness.* New York and London: Thomson Texere, 2004.

United States Agency for Healthcare Research Quality. "National Guidelines Clearinghouse." http: //www.guideline.gov.

Van Fraassen, B. *The Scientific Image.* New York: Oxford University Press, 1980.

Wightman, W. *The Emergence of Scientific Medicine.* Edinburgh: Oliver and Boyd, 1971.

## CHAPTER THREE

American Association for Clinical Chemistry Cardiac Risk Assessment. http://www.labtestsonline.org/understanding/analytes/cardiac_risk/glance.html.

Beckett, N., et al. "Treatment of Hypertension in Patients 80 Years of Age or Older." *New England Journal of Medicine* 358 (2008): 1887–98.

Best, J. *Damned Lies and Statistics*. Los Angeles: University of California Press, 2001.

Hildreth, C.J., A.E. Burke, and R.M. Glass. "JAMA Patient Page: Risk Factors for Heart Disease." *Journal of the American Medical Association* 27 (2009): 2176.

Walker, A.M. *Observation and Inference: An Introduction to the Methods of Epidemiology*. Chestnut Hill, MA: Epidemiology Resources Inc., 1991.


## CHAPTER FOUR

Dorner, B. "Promoting an Easier Swallow." *Provider* 28 (2002): 69–70.

Gupta, V., and L.A. Lipsitz. "Orthostatic Hypotension in the Elderly: Diagnosis and Treatment." *American Journal of Medicine* 120 (2007): 841–47.

Hollman, C. "Applying Sound Principles of Nutrition in Nursing Homes." *Nursing Older People* 13 (2001): 37.


## CHAPTER FIVE

Campbell, H., et al. "Integrated Care Pathways." *British Medical Journal* 316 (1998): 133–37.

Graf, C. "Functional Decline in Hospitalized Older Adults." *American Journal of Nursing* 106 (2006): 58–67.

Mendelsohn, R.S. *Confessions of a Medical Heretic*. Chicago: Contemporary Books, 1979.

Richards, J.R., and S.J. Ferrall. "Inappropriate Use of Emergency Medical Services Transport: Comparison of Provider and Patient Perspectives." *Academic Emergency Medicine* 6 (1999): 14–20.

Schneiderman, L.J., M.S. Jecker, and A.R. Jonsen. "Medical Futility: Its Meaning and Ethical Implications." *Annals of Internal Medicine* 112 (1990): 949–54.

Thomas, E.J., and T.A. Brennan. "Incidence and Types of Preventable Adverse Events in Elderly Patients: Population Based Review of Medical Records." *British Medical Journal* 320 (2000): 741–44.


## CHAPTER SIX

Gravelle, H., et al. "Impact of Case Management (Evercare) on Frail Elderly Patients: Controlled Before and After Analysis of Quantitative Outcome Data." *British Medical Journal* 334 (2007): 31.

Matter, C.A., et al. "Hospital to Home: Improving Internal Medicine Residents' Understanding of the Needs of Older Persons after a Hospital Stay." *Academic Medicine* 78 (2003): 793–97.

Nay, R. "Contradictions between Perceptions and Practices of Caring in Long-Term Care of Elderly People." *Journal of Clinical Nursing* 7 (1998): 401–8.

Pulsford, D., and J. Duxbury. "Aggressive Behaviour by People with Dementia in Residential Care Settings: A Review." *Journal of Psychiatric & Mental Health Nursing* 13 (2006): 611–18.


## CHAPTER SEVEN

Centers for Medicare and Medicaid Services. *National Health Expenditure Projections, 2006–2016*. Baltimore: U.S. Department of Health and Human Services, Centers for Medicare and Medicaid Services, 2007.

Henry J. Kaiser Family Foundation. *Health Care Costs: A Primer*. Menlo Park, CA: Henry J. Kaiser Family Foundation, 2007.

Jones, S. *Demographic Trends in America: Squaring the Population Pyramid*. Washington, DC: Washington Forum, 1987.

National PACE Association. http://www.npaonline.org.

Provincial and Territorial Ministers of Health. *Understanding Canada's Health Care Costs: Final Report*. Provincial and Territorial Ministers of Health, 2000.

**CHAPTER EIGHT**

Berger, J. "Pharmaceutical Industry Influences on Physician Prescribing: Gifts, Quasi-gifts, and Patient-Directed Gifts." *The American Journal of Bioethics* 3 (2003): 56–57.

Illich, I. *Medical Nemesis: The Expropriation of Health.* New York: Pantheon, 1976.

Moynihan, R., and A. Cassels. *Selling Sickness: How the World's Biggest Pharmaceutical Companies Are Turning Us All into Patients.* Vancouver: Greystone Books/New York: Nation, 2005.

Pfizer Inc. http: //www.pfizer.com.

Sloan, J., et al. "A Pilot Study of Anabolic Steroids in Elderly Patients with Hip Fractures." *Journal of the American Geriatric Society* 40 (1992): 1105–11.


**CHAPTER NINE**

Exton-Smith, A. "Terminal Illness in the Aged." *Lancet* II (1961): 305–8.

Kafetz, K. "What Happens When Elderly People Die?" *Journal of the Royal Society of Medicine* 95 (2002): 536–38.

Kübler-Ross, E. *On Death and Dying.* New York: Macmillan, 1970.

Kuhl, D. *What Dying People Want.* New York: Public Affairs, 2002.

Nicolaides-Bouman, A., et al. "Home Visiting Programme for Older People with Health Problems: Process Evaluation." *Journal of Advanced Nursing* 58 (2007): 425–35.

Nishimura, A., et al. "Patients Who Complete Advance Directives and What They Prefer." *Mayo Clinic Proceedings* 82 (2007): 1480–86.

Sloan, J. "Advance Directives: Patient Preferences in Family Practice." *Canadian Family Physician* 36 (1990): 876–78.

**CHAPTER TEN**

Bridges, B. *Therapeutic Caregiving: A Practical Guide for Caregivers of Persons with Alzheimer's Disease and Other Dementia-Causing Diseases.* Mill Creek, WA: BJB Publishing, 1995.

Loverde, J. *The Complete Eldercare Planner: Where to Start, Questions to Ask, and Where to Find Help.* New York: Hyperion, 1997.

Munsch, R., *Love You Forever.* Scarborough, ON: Firefly, 1986.

Silin, P. *Nursing Homes: The Family's Journey.* London and Baltimore: Johns Hopkins, 2001.

# Index

Personal names are fictionalized in some case studies.

academic doctors. *See* medical research and researchers
Ackerman, Mitchell (case study), 96–98, 106–7
advance directives, 191–94, 232–33
Alzheimer's disease, 21
angina, 62–64, 88
Arnesen, Helen (case study), 207–8, 223
arthritis, 21, 228–29
aspirin, for blood thinning, 66
atrial fibrillation, 66
autonomic nervous system, and blood pressure, 86–87

baby boomers, 139–41, 152–53, 156
bed sores, 96–98
Bellamy, Margaret (case study), 34–35
best practice, 64–65, 167, 221. *See also* clinical guidelines
blood pressure, high, 64–66, 78, 94, 229. *See also* hypertension in the very elderly trial
blood pressure, low: as cause of drowsiness, 14–15; causes of, 61–62, 85, 89, 236; dangers of, 84–90, 199–200; diet and, 83–84; as heart attack symptom, 33, 111–12

Boisvert, Henri (case study), 118–19, 127–29, 131
"burden" problem, 181–82, 195, 198, 203–4, 218, 233–35. *See also* dependence

cardiac arrest resuscitation, 190, 193
caregivers and caregiving, 211–35; accepting death, 217–18; communication and honesty, 208, 212, 215–16, 218; companionship, 220–21, 223; difficult patients, 204; drug evaluation guidelines, 229–30; hospitalized patients, 219–20; individuality of patient, 216–17, 221–22; model for home care, 222–35; needs and limitations, 122, 222–25; paid care providers, 225–26; pain control, 218–19. *See also* "burden" problem; dependence; primary care
Cassels, Alan, 158, 163
Chau, Mrs. (case study), 110–12, 185–86
cholesterol, 68–69, 78
Cleaver, Martha (case study), 98–99, 108–9, 113
Clinical Frailty Scale, 18–19
clinical guidelines: diagnosis and, 57–58; drugs and, 141, 177–78; in hospital, 105–8; limitations of, 102; in malpractice lawsuits, 56; vs. primary care responsibility, 173–75; risk states and, 78–79; set by academic leaders, 168–69;

triggered by tests, 85–86; uniformity of, 54–55

cognitive ability. *See* dementia; mental ability

comfort, as priority for fragile elderly, 27–28, 30–31, 113–14, 193–94, 229. *See also* pain

common sense, 67–69, 81, 202

communication: between caregivers and fragile elderly, 212, 215–16, 218; between emergency responders and family doctors, 103–4; gaps in discharge plans, 125–26; between home care workers and family doctors, 120–21; honesty in, 212, 215–16, 218, 222, 231–35

*Confessions of a Medical Heretic* (Mendelsohn), 105

congestive heart failure: case studies, 61–62, 111–12; clinical guidelines, 173; diagnosis of, 57–58; as risk state, 78; treatment of, 85, 228–29

consistency and reliability, 54–56, 58–59, 174, 176–77, 178–79. *See also* clinical guidelines

crisis: vs. death with dignity, 185–86, 187; decisions about, 193; emergency response to, 144–46, 147–48; of function, vs. dangerous illness, 23, 26–27, 101–2, 108–14, 144; rescue from, 217

critical care. *See* rescue (acute and critical care)

Crow, Harriet (case study), 149–50

daily function: and dependence, 21–22; drugs for, 30–31, 229; as priority for fragile elderly, 23, 24–25; sequence of collapse, 22; support of, in crises, 109–10, 217

Darren (case study), 64–65

Davenport, Ann (case study), 181–82

Davidson, Chuck (case study), 206–7, 215

death and dying: advance directives, 191–94, 232–33; attitudes toward, 35–37, 181–83, 189–91; deterioration and crisis, 185–86; with dignity, 185, 186–89; in hospitals, 105, 112–14; models of, 184–85; predictability of, 187; proximity of, 33–37

dehydration, 61–62, 88–89, 91–92

delirium, 91–92, 187

dementia: agitated and combative patients, 128–32; case studies, 116–19, 146, 209; vs. drug side effects, 81; effects on functioning, 21; and informed consent, 74–75

dependence, 17, 21–24, 35, 119. *See also* "burden" problem

depression, 30, 69–70, 194–95, 219

De Voord, Hannah (case study), 144–46, 150–51

Dhalliwal, Indrjit (case study), 209–10

diabetes, 49–51, 57, 78, 85, 94–95

diagnosis: of agitated patients, 129; and clinical guidelines, 57–58, 78–79; deceptive symptoms, 88; of heart disease, 57–58, 85; in hospital emergency rooms, 103; as primary care responsibility, 131, 173; uncertainty in, 112–13, 209

diet and nutrition, 82–84, 89, 92–95

discharge planning, 124–26

disease definitions. *See* diagnosis

diuretics, 61–62

Drug Benefit Committee, 160

drug industry, 52–53, 158, 160–68, 170–72, 177–78

drug payment plans, 138–39, 141–42, 160

drugs: for angina, 63–64; for blood thinning, 66; for cholesterol, 68–69; for comfort and daily functioning, 30–31; for dementia, 118–19; diuretics, 61–62; effects on blood pressure, 62, 85, 89–90, 236; evaluation of, by users, 165–66; guidelines for family caregivers, 229–30; for heart failure, 61–62; and kidney function, 28–29; and liver function, 29; non-specific side effects of, 79–81; for osteoporosis prevention,

67; overmedication, 118–19; for pain, 188–89; for Parkinson's disease, 14–15; preventive, 39–40, 70–71, 142–44, 165–66; selective drugectomy, 230, 236–37; side effects of, 79–81, 228–29; textbook treatments for the fragile elderly, 40–41; unpredictable responses to, 31–33, 75–76, 227–29; useless drugs, 164–66. See also randomized controlled trials
Dunlop, Maggie (case study), 194–95

Eichel, Hannah (case study), 200–201
Einstein, Albert, 40, 45
elderly, defined, 17–18
emergency response and care, 101–4, 145–51. See also rescue (acute and critical care)
end-of-life care. See death and dying; palliative care
epidemiology, 41–42, 46–48, 51–52, 68–69, 228. See also randomized controlled trials
evidence-based health care, 42–43, 51–54, 75, 81, 102, 106. See also clinical guidelines; medical research and researchers

falls, 87, 88, 117, 199–200
falsifiability, 46–47, 48, 71–72, 228
family members. See caregivers and caregiving
Fedoruk, Nellie (case study), 48–51
fragile elderly, defined, 18, 19–29, 212–13
frailty, defined, 17, 18–19
function. See daily function

Gadsen, Henry, 158
Gorton, Ellen (case study), 13–14, 22–23

Halstadt, Dick (case study), 60–62, 88–89
Hamaguchi, Frank (case study), 199–200
Hauptmann, Guenter (case study), 15–16, 23, 26

heart attack: vs. angina, 88; best practice, 85; as cause of death, 190; diagnosis of, 57–58; symptoms, 33, 39–40, 111–12
heart disease: angina, 62–64, 88; blood pressure and, 229; cholesterol and, 68–69; diagnosis of, 57–58, 85; heart attack, 33, 39–40, 57–58, 85, 88, 111–12, 190. See also congestive heart failure
heart failure. See congestive heart failure
heterogeneity: as characteristic of fragile elderly, 28–31, 58; in diabetes management, 50–51; in drug responses, 31–33, 75–76, 227–29; in epidemiology, 47–48; in symptoms, 31–33. See also individualized medicine
Higgins, Dorothy (case study), 135
home support: comfort in, 113–14; communication by doctors, 120–21; costs of, vs. hospital care, 98; limits of responsibility, 120–21; minor surgery, 146–48; vs. rescue, 101–4, 112, 114, 145–46; value of, for fragile elderly, 123–24. See also caregivers and caregiving; primary care
honesty. See communication
hospitals, 96–115; admission decisions, 98, 108–14; appropriate for fragile elderly, 209–10, 216; bed sores, treatment of, 96–98; clinical guidelines and pathways, 105–6, 107–8; death in, 98–99, 105, 112–14, 190; discharge plans, 124–26; as elder-sitting services, 149–50; errors as system breakdown, 158–59; fear of, 98; inappropriate for the fragile elderly, 99–103, 154–56, 196–97, 219–20; limits of responsibility, 121–22; loss of identity in, 196; morale in, 196–98; and multiple pathology, 104; nosocomial infections, 97–98; psychiatric assessment, 97–98; risk management in, 107; as substitute for home care, 96–98, 121, 149–50
Hume, David, 45, 46
hypertension in the very elderly trial, 74, 77, 89

hypoglycemia, 49–50. *See also* diabetes

Illich, Ivan, 158–59, 172, 215
individualized medicine: vs. epidemiology, 51–52; non-falsifiability of, 71–72; vs. prevention and rescue, 75–76, 216–17, 221–22; vs. randomized controlled trials, 53; as science, 201–2; teaching of, 55. *See also* primary care
infections: as functional crises, 26, 80, 109, 191; as serious crises, 112–13, 145
influenza, variation with age, 34–35
informed consent, 74–75

Kalinska, Elzbieta (case study), 182–83, 203
kidney function, 28–29, 98–99
Kübler-Ross, Elisabeth, 184, 185
Kuhl, David, 186

liver function, variation with age, 29
living wills. *See* advance directives
loneliness. *See* social isolation
*Love You Forever* (Munsch), 234

malpractice, 56, 127, 158
Martin, Emily (case study), 187–89
McCarthy, Mary (case study), 5–6, 236–37
McKenzie, Howard (case study), 14–15, 23
media, health reporting by, 42–44
medical administrators, 134–35, 154–56, 175–79
medical education, 161–63, 171
medical ethics, 53, 73–75, 166–67
*Medical Nemesis* (Illich), 158–59, 172, 215
medical research and researchers, 168–72. *See also* epidemiology; randomized controlled trials
medical system, 134–57; administrative guidelines, 176–78; baby boomers in, 139–40, 152–53, 156; disproportionate expenditures for fragile elderly, 141–44; fragile elderly as outliers, 58; home support initiatives, 155–57;

morale of health care workers, 196–98; prevention and rescue as priorities, 41, 137–38; resources wasted on fragile elderly, 138–39, 153–55, 221; successes of, 42–43. *See also* emergency response and care; hospitals; "prevention and rescue" model of medicine
Mendelsohn, Robert, 105
mental ability, 97–98, 107, 193. *See also* dementia
Meredith, Gwyn (case study), 82–84, 93
mobility impairment, 21–22, 80
morale, of health care workers, 196–98
Morales, Victor (case study), 190–91
Moynihan, Ray, 158, 163
multiple pathology, 20–21, 73–75, 78–79, 103–4, 164
Munsch, Robert, 234

Neall, Daisy (case study), 91–92
Newton, Isaac, 45, 47
NIMBYism, in geriatric care, 116–33; case studies, 116–19, 123–24, 127–32; communication problems, 120–21; community support, 121; and hospital discharge, 123–27; hospital limitations, 121–22; responsibility, denial of, 122–23
nosocomial infections, 97–98
nursing homes, 92, 94–95, 129–32, 225. *See also* caregivers and caregiving
nutrition. *See* diet and nutrition

O'Malley, Elizabeth (case study), 39–41, 196
On Lok Lifeways, 156
orthorexia, 93
osteoporosis, 57, 67, 78, 90, 229

pain: and depression, 194–95; drugs for, 30, 194–95; effects of, 21–22; in Parkinson's disease, 188–89; prevention of, 198, 204, 218–19. *See also* comfort, as priority for fragile elderly
palliative care, 36–37, 184–85, 186

Parkinson's disease, 14–15, 31, 187–89
polymyalgia rheumatica, 186
Popper, Karl, 45–46, 71
population age structure, 139–41,
    152–53, 156
predictability, in science and epidemiol-
    ogy, 47–48. *See also* heterogeneity
pressure sores, 96–98
"prevention and rescue" model of medi-
    cine, 41, 137–38; vs. comfort, 193–94;
    identifying when to abandon it, 17,
    119–20, 214–15; reorientation of, for
    fragile elderly, 184, 217–18. *See also*
    preventive medicine; rescue (acute and
    critical care)
preventive medicine, 64–81, 82–96; age-
    specific benefits, 66–67; age-specific
    research, 72–75; case studies, 60–64,
    82–84, 91–92; clinical guidelines, 78–
    79; vs. comfort and daily functioning,
    25, 218–19; common sense in, 67–69,
    81; difficult to observe effects, 70–71;
    drugs for, 70–71, 142–44; inappropriate
    for the fragile elderly, 229; individuals
    and risk statistics, 75–78; overmedica-
    tion, 79–81; risks of, 61–62; useless
    drugs for, 165–66. *See also* blood pres-
    sure, low; diet and nutrition; drugs
primary care: big-picture responsibil-
    ity, 132–33; blamed for problems of
    fragile elderly, 172–75; choice of doctor,
    229–31; at home, 7–8, 157, 214, 226–27;
    on-call demands and gaps in care,
    129–32; vs. rescue, 122; standard
    model of, 120
professional care providers, 196–98,
    225–31. *See also* hospitals; primary care
Program of All-inclusive Care of the
    Elderly (PACE), 156
publication bias, 169–70
pulmonary embolism, 98–99

randomized controlled trials: correla-
    tions vs. cause, 68–69; as evidence
base, 52–54; falsifiability in, 71–72;
    fragile elderly excluded from, 53,
    72–75; hypertension in the very elderly
    trial, 74, 77, 89; informed consent,
    74–75; medical ethics in, 166–67; in
    preventive medicine, 71, 72. *See also*
    epidemiology; medical research and
    researchers
reliability. *See* consistency and reliability
rescue (acute and critical care), 96–115;
    appropriate use of, 137–38; availability
    of, 102–3; case studies, 96–99; in crises
    of fragile elderly, 26, 101–4, 108–15;
    vs. home support, 112, 114, 145–46;
    hospitals as traps for the fragile
    elderly, 104–6; limitations of, 121–22;
    vs. primary care, 122; rigidity of, 101–2.
    *See also* emergency response and care;
    hospitals
responsibility: as contract, 233–34; dis-
    cussions about, 233–35; of families and
    caregivers, 213–15; vs. fragmented care,
    127–32, 226–27; honesty, 215–16; in pri-
    mary care, 173–75. *See also* NIMBYism,
    in geriatric care
risk management, 61–62, 76–78, 107
risk states, 72–73, 78–79
Rockwood, Kenneth, 18–19

Scarlatti, Dave (case study), 62–64, 88
Schoenfeld, Emil (case study), 182
science: applied to health of fragile
    elderly, 67, 159, 199, 201–2, 211, 228;
    assumptions of, 58; as gold standard,
    41–42, 44–47; nutrition research, 93–
    94. *See also* epidemiology; falsifiability;
    medical research and researchers;
    randomized controlled trials
selective drugectomy, 230, 236–37
*Selling Sickness* (Cassels & Moynihan),
    158, 163
senses (taste and smell), 88–89, 93
Seppanen, Kirsti (case study),
    116–18, 123–24

social isolation, 198–202, 205, 220
strokes: effects of, 21, 186–87; prevention
  of, 65–66, 69, 74, 77; symptoms of, 33
support groups and respite, 224
surgery, 15, 91, 145, 146–48, 151
swallowing disorders, 90–92

Taleb, Nassim, 40, 50
Thompson, Delbert (case study), 146–48

urinary tract infections, 33, 118–19

wait times, 138
weakness, 22
*What Dying People Want* (Kuhl), 186
wishes and goals of the fragile elderly,
  181–205; end-of-life care, 183–89;
  freedom from pain and intolerable symptoms, 188–89, 194–95, 198,
  204; meaningful relationships and
  company, 183, 198–202, 203, 205;
  milestones, 190–91; not to be a burden,
  181–82, 195, 198, 203–4, 218, 233–35; not
  to be resuscitated, 190, 192–93; not to
  miss anything, 182; self-respect and
  identity, 183, 196, 198, 204; to be listened to, 191, 205. *See also* hospitals

## About the Author

JOHN SLOAN, MD, is a senior academic physician in the Department of Family Practice at the University of British Columbia and has spent most of his thirty years of practice caring for the frail elderly. He lives in Vancouver and Roberts Creek, British Columbia.